THE UNIVERSITY OF MICHIGAN MEDICAL CENTER PARENTERAL AND ENTERAL NUTRITION MANUAL

This manual has been prepared and edited by:

John R. Wesley, M.D.
Nabil Khalidi, Pharm.D.
Walter C. Faubion, M.S., R.N.
Debra S. Kovacevich, B.S.N., R.N.
Carol L. Braunschweig, M.S., R.D.
Christopher J. Maksym, Pharm.D.
Susan M. Revesz, M.S.N., R.N.
Anne M. Perez, B.S.N., R.N.
Debra D. Wilson, M.S., R.D.
Bessie Marikis, Pharm.D.
Arnold G. Coran, M.D.

D1738084

Acknowledgements

The Parenteral and Enteral Nutrition Team is grateful to all members of the Parenteral and Enteral Nutrition Steering Committee for their guidance and to the Department of Pharmacy Services for their support. The following individuals are acknowledged for their specific contributions in the development and review of this manual:

Robert W. Bartlett, M.D.
Robert Schumacher, M.D.
Ellen Kent, Secretary
Kelly Spitler, Secretary

Reviewed by the Pharmacy and Therapeutics Committee with the approval of the EXECUTIVE COMMITTEE on CLINICAL AFFAIRS, 1990.

PARENTERAL AND ENTERAL NUTRITION STEERING COMMITTEE MEMBERS

Name	Department	Phone
August, David, M.D.	Surgery	6-5783
Bartlett, Robert, M.D.	Surgery	6-5822
Bickley, Sue, Pharm.D.	Pharmacy	6-8986
Braunschweig, Carol, M.S, R.D.	PEN Team	6-8231
Brewer, Karolyn, R.N., M.S.	Home Care	4-0589
Coon, William, M.D.	Surgery	6-5814
Coran, Arnold, M.D.	Pediatric Surgery	4-4151
Custer, Joseph, M.D.	Pediatric ICU	3-5302
Dechert, Ronald, R.R.T., M.S.	Metabolic Lab	6-5860
Dickenson, Chris, M.D.	Pediatric— Gastroenterology	3-9650
Drewnowski, Adam, Ph.D.	School of Public Health	7-0208
Elta, Grace, M.D.	Internal Medicine— Gastroenterology	6-4780
Faubion, Walter M.S., R.N.	PEN Team	6-8233
Graham, Carol, B.S.N., R.N.	PEN Team	6-8233
Hutchinson, Raymond, M.D.	Pediatric Hematology— Oncology	4-7126
Ike, Robert, M.D.	Internal Medicine, Arthritis	6-5565
Kerestes-Smith, Joyce, R.D., M.S.	Dietetics	6-5189
Khalidi, Nabil, Pharm.D.	PEN Team	6-8223
Kovacevich, Debra, B.S.N., R.N.	PEN Team	6-8231
Lown, Debbie, R.D.	Dietetics	6-5921
Maksym, Chris, Pharm.D.	PEN Team	6-8231
Marikis, Bessie, Pharm.D.	PEN Team	6-8231
Mehta, Varsha, Pharm.D.	Pharmacy-Holden	6-8986
Nostrant, Timothy, M.D.	Internal Medicine— Gastroenterology	6-4775
Olson, Alan, M.D.	Pediatric— Gastroenterology	3-9650
Perez, Anne, B.S.N., R.N.	PEN Team	6-8231
Prasad, Jai, M.D.	Burn Unit	6-9631
Revesz, Susan, M.S.N., R.N.	PEN Team	6-8231
Rodriguez, Jorge, M.D.	Surgery	6-5797
Rosenblum, Lee, B.S.	Social Services	6-5963
Roskos, Rudolf, M.D.	Pediatrics	4-7126
Saran, Patricia, B.S.N., R.N.	Surgical Nursing	3-0286
Schumacher, Robert, M.D.	Neonatology	3-4109
Swartz, Richard, M.D.	Internal Medicine— Nephrology	6-4890
Thomson, Phil, Ph.D.	Burn Unit	6-9673
Wesley, John, M.D.	Pediatric Surgery, Chairman, PEN Team Steering Committee	4-6846
Wilson, Debra, M.S., R.D.	PEN Team	6-8231
Yonkoski, Debra, M.B.A., R.D.	Dietetics	6-5909

ORGANIZATIONAL CHART

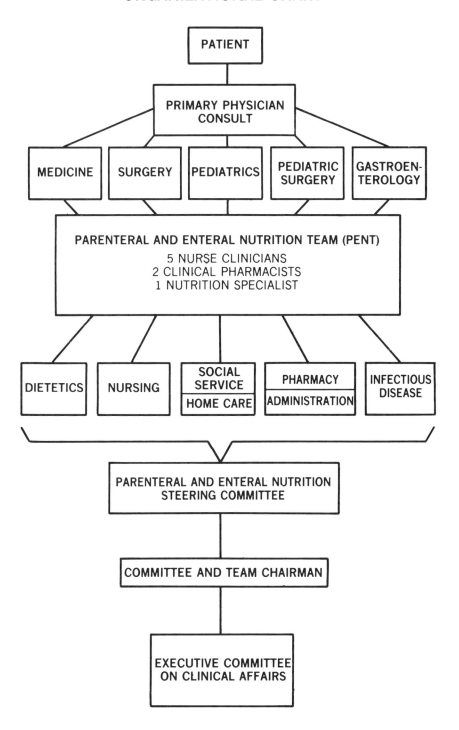

TABLE OF CONTENTS

I. INTRODUCTION

Optimal nutritional care of the hospitalized patient requires careful evaluation and trial of the large variety of diets available through the Departments of Pharmacy Services and Dietetics. When enteral feedings are impossible or inadequate in meeting the patient's nutritional requirements, the physician must turn to parenteral nutrition, either supplementary or total, to supply the patient's metabolic needs. This manual is not intended to be a textbook on nutrition; rather it is intended to provide guidelines for the evaluation and management of patients with exceptional nutritional requirements.

Definition

Total parenteral nutrition (TPN) is the administration of complete nutrition by intravenous infusion in order to maintain or restore body weight and an anabolic state when oral or enteral routes are not feasible. Parenteral nutrition (PN) may be administered by central or peripheral vein using a hyperosmolar solution according to the patient's needs and underlying disease process.

II. PARENTERAL AND ENTERAL NUTRITION (PEN) TEAM AND STEERING COMMITEE

A. Organization

When used properly, total parenteral nutrition is beneficial to the patient and even lifesaving. When used improperly, it is hazardous, even life threatening, with many reported infections and mechanical complications. For these reasons, a Parenteral and Enteral Nutrition (PEN) Team was authorized by The Executive Committee on Clinical Affairs of the University of Michigan Medical Center in December 1978, to establish and maintain patient care guidelines in this rapidly changing field.

The University of Michigan Medical Center Parenteral and Enteral Nutrition Steering Committee consists of resident and staff members from the following disciplines: General Surgery, Pediatric Surgery, Internal Medicine, Pediatric and Adult Oncology, Pediatrics, Neonatology, Pediatric and Adult Gastroenterology, Infectious Disease, Nursing, Pharmacy, Dietetics, Social Services, and Home Care. The Steering Committee is responsible to The Executive Committee on Clinical Affairs through its elected Chairman and meets monthly. The committee has hired a core team consisting of five Nurse Clinicians, two Clinical Pharmacists, and one Nutrition Specialist. Their main functions are to provide expert advice and patient care monitoring.

B. General Goals

The general goals of the Steering Committee and Team are to establish hospital wide guidelines and protocols intended to maximize patient benefits from parenteral and enteral nutrition while minimizing the potential complications, and to exchange new ideas such that the recommended guidelines will reflect the most current data and best therapeutic judgment available.

C. Specific Goals

The many advantages of the team approach to the management of patients requiring special parenteral and enteral nutrition have been summarized in a number of publications. The specific goals of the Parenteral and Enteral Nutrition Team are to provide:

1. A source of expertise available for consultation by specialty and general services to help determine the indications for parenteral nutrition for any given patient.
2. Guidelines for daily orders on patients receiving parenteral nutrition.
3. Formal instruction of nurses and house staff in the fundamentals and techniques of parenteral nutrition.
4. Quality control in the form of scheduled rounds to check the apparatus and techniques of administering parenteral nutrition.
5. Advice and supervision during the transition period from parenteral nutrition (PN) to oral alimentation or tube feeding (enteral nutrition).
6. Instruction and supervision of patients and families involved in the preparation and administration of parenteral and/or enteral nutrition at home.
7. Continuing education regarding new developments in parenteral nutrition for medical and other hospital staff at all levels.
8. Reduction in the incidence of catheter sepsis and other PN related complications.
9. A system for collection and review of data on intra-hospital parenteral nutrition utilization and cost-effectiveness.

III. CONSULTATION PROCEDURE FOR PATIENTS RECEIVING PN

All patients receiving PN will be seen on a scheduled basis by one or more members of the core team (five nurse clinicians, two clinical pharmacists, and one nutrition specialist). This service will commence automatically when Pharmacy receives the first set of orders for PN. No formal consultation need be written for this quality assurance service.

If a physician desires a formal consultation concerning the indications for PN, setting up a regimen for PN, or specific metabolic nutritional problems with respect to a patient, he may consult any member of the PEN Team or Steering Committee individually (see inside front cover). The mechanics for consultation are exactly the same as for every other hospital consultation with respect to filling out the consultation form and calling the service or individual requested. If a physician does not know which member of the team to consult for a particular patient problem, he may call the PEN Team office (telephone number 6-8231) or page a PEN Team member directly.

	Page No.
Manager	2479
Clinical Pharmacists	2940, 2475
Nurse Clinician (Pediatric)	1361
Nurse Clinicians (Adult)	2476, 2477, 1362
Nutrition Specialist	2927
Nutrition Specialist (Holden)	0766

IV. NUTRITIONAL ASSESSMENT

Nutritional assessment should be a fundamental part of the basic workup for a hospitalized patient and should be completed prior to implementing enteral or parenteral nutrition. Severe malnourishment is usually easily recognized. However, patients in a state of moderate malnourishment are a challenge to the health professional's diagnostic skills. Malnourished patients have impaired wound healing, compromised immune status, and a higher incidence of morbidity and mortality. Early identification of patients at risk of progressing into severe nutritional depletion is the first step in providing proper nutritional therapy. Establishing simple baseline nutritional parameters, such as height, weight, albumin, and transferrin, provide direction for nutritional management. A complete nutritional assessment should include evaluation of risk factors, diet history, clinical examination, laboratory data, energy requirements, and in some instances, anthropometric measurements. The patient's nutritional status should be reviewed weekly throughout the hospital stay and treatment plans revised accordingly.

A. Risk Factors

The following factors denote the presence of, or risk of developing, some degree of protein-calorie malnutrition (PCM). Absence of these characteristics is not a guarantee that malnutrition does not exist or will not occur.

1. Usual body weight 20% above or below ideal weight.
2. Recent loss of 10% or more of usual body weight.
3. Excessive alcohol intake.
4. Chronic disease.
5. NPO for more than 7 days on intravenous solutions for hydration.
6. Increased metabolic needs:
   a. Extensive burns, trauma, surgery
   b. Protracted fever, infection
   c. Draining abscesses, wounds, fistulas
   d. Pregnancy
   e. Prematurity of infants
7. Protracted nutrient losses:
   a. Malabsorption syndromes
   b. Short gut syndrome
   c. Draining abscesses, wounds, fistulas
   d. Renal dialysis
   e. Effusions
   f. Chronic blood loss
8. Intake of drugs with catabolic effects:
   a. Steroids
   b. Immunosuppressants
   c. Antitumor agents
9. Protracted emesis associated with:
   a. Anorexia
   b. Pregnancy
   c. Radiation or chemotherapy
   d. Obstruction

B. Diet History

A detailed diet history is important in assessing a patient's nutritional status. A clinical dietitian may be contacted to help obtain an accurate history, assess baseline status, and detect subclinical deficiencies or toxicities. Changes in taste, appetite, intake, weight, or consumption of a special diet may indicate a significantly altered nutritional status. Dentition, finances, level of independence, sociocultural background and level of nutritional education should also be assessed.

C. Clinical Examination

The clinical manifestation of malnutrition may vary greatly in specificity and severity. Vitamin and mineral deficiencies are frequently associated with malnutrition. Although classic far-advanced symptoms are occasionally encountered, symptoms of vitamin deficiencies are often mild, nonspecific, and may be signs of non-nutritional abnormalities. Therefore, physical findings of malnutrition must be interpreted in light of the patient's history.

Normal body weight or obesity are not guarantees of adequate nutritional status. When discussing calorie and/or protein malnutrition, two terms are important to define. Acute malnutrition (Kwashiorkor) describes malnutrition in the protein-depleted patient with adequate fat stores. A typical hospitalized patient suffering from acute malnutrition might be obese while under stress. Chronic malnutrition (Marasmus) represents depletion of both protein and fat stores. This is the classic emaciated-appearing, malnourished patient. A patient with chronic malnutrition generally has a long history of poor oral intake and is not hypermetabolic.

Both acute and chronic malnutrition represent severe nutritional deficiencies (Table 1). Most hospitalized patients will be somewhere between the two extremes.

TABLE 1

Protein-Calorie Malnutrition (Marasmus)	Acute Protein Malnutrition (Kwashiorkor)
Visceral proteins may be maintained (Albumin & Transferrin)	Visceral proteins depleted
Somatic protein depleted	Somatic protein depleted
Body fat stores depleted	Normal or increased body fat (flabby)
Emaciated, "skin and bones" appearance	Normal or increased body weight
Edema not usually present	Edema
Sparse, dry, easily plucked hair	Sparse, dry, easily plucked hair in severe cases
Delayed wound healing	Delayed wound healing

D. Evaluation of Nutritional Status

The recommended assessment parameters, to evaluate nutritional status and support are included in Table 2. In addition to these parameters, a detailed description of diet history and anthropometrics are provided in the Physician's Handbook of Nutrition Support. A copy of this manual is located in each patient unit.

E. Estimation of Nutritional Requirements

1. Energy Requirements

   a. Estimation

   Basal energy expenditure (BEE) refers to the metabolic activity required to maintain life, i.e. respiration, heart beat, maintenance of body temperature and other essential functions. The BEE can be estimated using the Harris-Benedict equation described below:

   For men $BEE = 66 + (13.7 \times W) + (5 \times H) - (6.8 \times A)$
   For women $BEE = 655 + (9.6 \times W) + (1.7 \times H) - (4.7 \times A)$

   W = Actual weight in kilograms
   H = Height in centimeters
   A = Age in years

   Resting energy expenditure (REE) is approximately 10% higher than BEE because it adjusts for the thermic effect of food and an awake state.

   Total energy expenditure is estimated by multiplying the BEE by the appropriate factor as indicated below:

   Maintenance
      Bedrest $1.2 \times BEE$
      Ambulatory $1.3 \times BEE$
      Anabolic $1.5 \times BEE$
      Stress/Starvation $1.2 \times BEE \times$ percent change in metabolic activity

   Figure 1 provides a nomogram for determination of the % change in metabolic activity.

   Energy requirements should also be increased 12% with each degree of fever above 37 degrees C.

   Figures 2, 3, and Table 3 provide alternate methods for estimating energy requirements using a series of nomograms.

   b. Measurement of Energy Expenditure

   Resting energy expenditure (REE) is determined by measuring oxygen consumption (VO_2) in a resting steady state. If VO_2 stays reasonably constant over 24 hours, once a day measurements can be extrapolated to 24 hour periods.

   VO_2 can be measured in two ways:

   1. Inspired — expired gas analysis or volumetric spirometry (Accuracy $\pm$ 5%)

2. Fick Equation — (Accuracy ± 15%)

VO_2 = Cardiac output x AVO_2 difference

AVO_2 difference = arterial minus venous O_2 content

Venous O_2 content = Hgb x venous O_2 Sat x 1.36

Arterial O_2 content = Hgb x Arterial O_2 Sat x 1.36

REE = VO_2 L/min x 5 kcal/L* x 60 min/hr x 24 hr/day

*5 kcal/L = caloric equivalent of one L oxygen

Energy expenditure measurements can be obtained by contacting the Critical Care Diagnostic Service at 936-5860 (Dr. Robert Bartlett—Adults, Dr. John Wesley—Pediatrics)

2. Protein Requirements

a. Estimation

Protein needs should be determined using a patient's ideal body weight (IBW), which is a theoretical estimate based on height and frame size.

Tables 4 and 5 provide guidelines for estimation of IBW. The following factors can be used to estimate protein requirements:

Maintenance	0.8 — 1.0 g/kg IBW
Repletion	1.0 — 1.5 g/kg IBW
Renal Failure	0.5 — 1.5 g/kg IBW (adjust for chronic and acute failure and dialysis)
Liver Failure	0.5 — 0.6 g/kg IBW (initially, then increase as tolerated)

3. Fluid Requirements

a. Maintenance of basal fluid requirements can be estimated as follows:

100 mL/kg for the first 10 kg of body weight
50 mL/kg for the second 10 kg of body weight
20 mL/kg for each kg of body weight over 20 kg

For every degree increase in body temperature above 38 degrees C, approximately 10% more fluid above maintenance should be administered.

F. Evaluation of Nutritional Support Therapy

Once the nutritional assessment is completed and nutrition support has begun, nutritional efficacy can be evaluated by serial measurements of transferrin, nitrogen balance and weight change. Additional measurements of nutritional repletion include wound healing, muscle strength, and improved respiratory parameters. Table 2 outlines the method for transferrin extrapolation from TIBC levels and the calculation of a standard nitrogen balance.

1. Interpretation of nitrogen balance data

   Nitrogen balance is the generally accepted method for evaluation of adequacy of protein intake. This technique is based on the premise that equilibrium in the adult is attained when the supply of protein is adequate to replace losses via the kidneys, intestinal secretions, sweat and desquamation of epithelial cells.

   Nitrogen balance is defined as:

   Nitrogen Balance = Nitrogen in − Nitrogen out

   $$\text{Nitrogen in} = \frac{\text{grams Protein intake from all sources}}{6.25}$$

   Protein catabolism (nitrogen out) is determined by measuring the excretion or accumulation of nitrogenous metabolic end products, particularly urea. In patients with normal renal function most of the nitrogen loss is in the urine with 80% of the nitrogen present as urea. Protein catabolism is calculated as:

   Nitrogen excreted = gm Nitrogen in 24 hr urine collection
   (accuracy ± 2%)

   or

   gm Urea Nitrogen in 24 hr urine collection
   (accuracy ± 20%)

   Protein catabolism (gm/day) = gm N/24 hr x 6.25 gmP

   If the patient is in renal failure protein catabolic rate is estimated as follows:

   PCR = Urine N_2 + Dialysate or filtrate N_2 + Urea accumulation

   Urea accumulation = B.U.N. mg/dl - baseline B.U.N. mg/dl x body wt (kg) x .6

Protein catabolic rates, nitrogen loss and nitrogen balance are made by the Critical Care Diagnostic Service: 936-5860

2. Limitations to nitrogen balance

   a. Nitrogen balance is the sum of total body gains and losses. Protein gains or losses of individual organs cannot be ascertained.

   b. In humans, adjustment to a nitrogen load occurs in a minimum of 3 to 5 days. To accurately assess adequacy or inadequacy of a nutrition support regimen, nitrogen balance should not be measured until a steady state is achieved.

   c. The constantly changing physiologic conditions of the ICU patient combined with constantly changing energy requirements makes nitrogen balance data very difficult to interpret as a measure of the adequacy or inadequacy of nutritional support. The nitrogen balance data in these patients should be used as a measure of their degree of catabolism and not necessarily the adequacy or inadequacy of protein intake. However, in general, it is desirable to achieve a positive nitrogen balance in these critically ill patients as soon as possible in keeping with appropriate physiologic principles.

TABLE 2
Degree of Impairment

Assessment Parameter	Normal	Degree of Impairment			Comments/Calculations/Limitations
		Mild	Moderate	Severe	
Time		Weight (% of change)			Should be done daily at the same time, on the same scale and with similar clothing. The average adult on full TPN is expected to gain 110-220 g/day (¼ - ½ lb) when the goal is repletion. $$\% \text{ weight loss} = \frac{\text{usual weight - current weight}}{\text{usual weight}} \times 100$$
1 week	—	0.5-1	1-2	>2	
1 mo	—	3-4	5	>5	
3 mo	—	6-7.0	7.5	>7.5	Limitation: Weight change may reflect increased or decreased hydration and not change in lean body mass. A weight loss of ≥5% within the preceding month indicates nutritional risk.
6 mo	—	8-9.5	10	>10	
Albumin, g%	≥3.5	3.5-3.0	3.0-2.5	<2.5	Albumin comprises over 50% of the visceral protein and has a half-life of 20 days. A serum level below 3.0 g% is associated with increased morbidity and mortality. Limitation: Due to long half-life of about 20 days, visceral depletion and repletion will not be detected rapidly. Serum levels may be affected by hepatic and renal disease, congestive heart failure and chronically draining wounds.
Transferrin, mg%	200-350	200-180	180-160	<160	Transferrin, a carrier protein involved in iron metabolism, is a more sensitive indicator of visceral protein deficit than albumin, since the half-life is approximately 9 days, and there is a smaller body pool. Limitation: Modified in the presence of infection, iron deficiency, hepatic and renal disease, congestive heart failure and chronically draining wounds. The specific conversion formula for the University of Michigan has been determined to be: transferrin = (TIBC × 0.66) + 42
Transthyretin (mg/dl) (Prealbumin)	>13	>10-13	10-6.5	<6.5	In conjunction with retinol binding protein, transthyretin transports retinol in the blood. The half life of transthyretin is approximately 2 days. It is synthesized within the hepatocyte. Limitation: levels are reduced in liver disease, after surgery, in sepsis and following trauma and thus do not reflect adequacy or inadequacy of nutritional status/support when these conditions are present.
Total Lymphocyte Count (TLC), cells/mm³	>1800	1800-1500	1500-900	<900	Provides a general guide to the patient's ability to respond to infection. Depressed in protein calorie malnutrition. $$\text{Total Lymphocyte Count} = \frac{\% \text{ lymphocytes} \times \text{WBC}}{100}$$ Limitation: Many factors other than PCM will cause a decrease in TLC, such as chemotherapy, sepsis and trauma.

TABLE 2 (Continued)

Assessment Parameter	Degree of Impairment				Comments/Calculations/Limitations
	Normal	Mild	Moderate	Severe	
Skin Test Antigens (mm)	>15	15-10	10-5	5-0	A test of cellular immune function. The test antigens are injected intradermally, and the area of induration (anergy) is measured in mm after 24 and 48 hours. Induration of 0-5 mm indicates failure of the patient to respond to foreign protein (anergy) or lack of previous exposure to antigen. Limitation: Factors other than malnutrition may suppress induration, such as chemotherapy, medications, and sepsis.
Urine Urea Nitrogen (UUN)					The values must be used in conjunction with the amount of nitrogen that has been administered and/or ingested and incorporated into a nitrogen balance profile. A 24 hour collection of urine is reported in grams of UUN excreted.
Nitrogen Balance					Repair of significant protein deficits can only occur if the nitrogen balance is significantly positive. Anabolism is indicated when (+) 4-5 g occurs. A near neutral or zero balance indicates that no change in the patient's nutritional status is likely to occur. If no deficit exists, maintaining zero nitrogen balance is desirable as a goal of therapy. A large negative nitrogen balance parallels a continuing and increasing deficit in the protein compartments. Reduction of 6.25 g total body protein occurs for each 1 g/day of negative nitrogen balance.

For the Skin Test Antigens:

Skin Test Antigen	Dilutions	Inject
Mumps	undiluted	0.1 mL
PPD	1:1000	0.1 mL
Candida albicans	10 PNU/mL	0.1 mL

For Nitrogen Balance:

ORAL AND ENTERAL INTAKE

$$\text{Protein intake in } \frac{g}{6.25} - N \text{ excreted or accumulated} = N \text{ Balance}$$

IV INTAKE

$$(gN/liter \times \#\ liters/day - (N\ out) = N\ Balance$$

IV AND ORAL INTAKE

$$(gN/liter \times \#\ liters/day) + \frac{\text{protein intake in } g}{6.25} - (N\ out) = \text{Nitrogen Balance}$$

N excretion should be directly measured. It can be estimated as UUN + 20%.

FIGURE 1
INDEX OF PERCENT CHANGE IN METABOLIC ACTIVITY

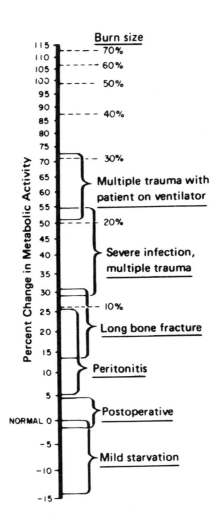

FIGURE 2
DETERMINATION OF SURFACE AREA FROM HEIGHT AND WEIGHT

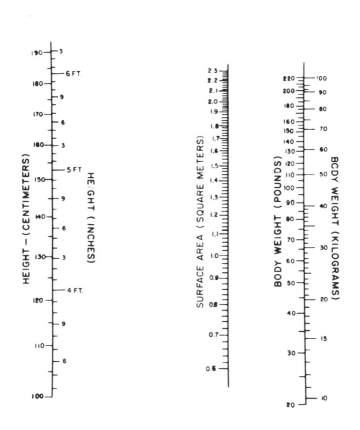

Figure 2: To determine body surface area from the height of the left-hand scale and weight on the right-hand scale, connect these points with a straightedge and read surface area from the middle scale.

TABLE 3
BASAL METABOLIC RATES FOR NORMALS

Age in Years	Males Kcal/m²/hr	Females Kcal/m²/hr
1	53	53
2-3	52	52
4-5	50	49
6-7	48	46
8-9	46	43
10-11	44	42
12-13	42	41
14-15	42	39
16-17	41	37
18-19	40	36
20-25	38	35
25-30	37	35
30-35	37	35
35-40	36	35
40-45	36	35
45-50	36	34
50-55	36	34
55-60	35	34
60-65	35	33
65-70	34	32
70-75	33	32
75 and over	33	31

FIGURE 3
PREDICTION OF DAILY BASAL METABOLIC RATE

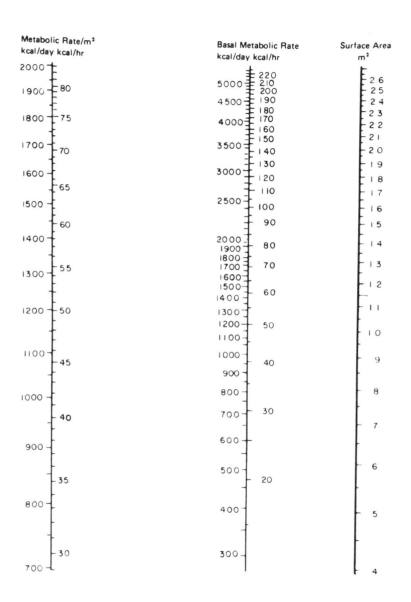

Figure 3: Determine surface area (Figure 2) and normal basal metabolic rate (Table 3). Connect these points with a straightedge. The predicted daily or hourly basal metabolic rate may then be determined from the middle scale. To account for the impact of a disease process, refer back to Figure 1.

TABLE 4

ESTIMATED WEIGHT ALLOWANCE FOR HEIGHT

Build	Women	Men
Medium	Allow 100 lb (45.5 kg) for first 5 ft (152 cm) of height plus 5 lb (2.3 kg) for each additional inch (2.5 cm)	Allow 106 lb (48 kg) for first 5 ft (152 cm) of height plus 6 lb (2.7 kg) for each additional inch (2.5 cm)
Small	Subtract 10%	Subtract 10%
Large	Add 10%	Add 10%

This table is reprinted from Committees of the American Diabetes Association, Inc. and The American Dietetic Association, 1977. *A guide for professionals: The effective application of exchange lists for meal planning*, p. 17.

Estimates of Frame Size*

Measure the wrist circumference just distal to the styloid process at the wrist crease of the right hand. Calculate the ratio (r) of body frame size to wrist circumference with the fomula:

$$r = \frac{H}{C}$$

where H = height in centimeters; C = wrist circumference in centimeters. Determine the frame size from the following table:

	r Value	
Frame Size	Men	Women
Small	>10.4	>10.9
Medium	10.4-9.6	10.9-9.9
Large	<9.6	<9.9

*Based on information provided in JP Grant, PB Custer, and J Thurlow: *Current techniques of nutritional assessment.* Surg Clin N Amer 61:437, 1981.

TABLE 5

STANDARDS FOR EVALUATION OF BODY WEIGHT

Fogarty International Center, Conference on Obesity: Desirable Weights for Heights and Ranges for Adult Males and Females

Height[a]		Recommended Weight for Men[b](lb)		Recommended Weight for Women[b](lb)	
Feet	Inches	Average	Range	Average	Range
4	10			102	92-119
4	11			104	94-122
5	0			107	96-125
5	1			110	99-128
5	2	123	112-141	113	102-131
5	3	127	115-144	116	105-134
5	4	130	118-148	120	108-138
5	5	133	121-152	123	111-142
5	6	136	124-156	128	114-146
5	7	140	128-161	132	118-150
5	8	145	132-166	136	122-154
5	9	149	136-170	140	126-158
5	10	153	140-174	144	130-163
5	11	158	144-179	148	134-168
6	0	162	148-184	152	138-173
6	1	166	152-189		
6	2	171	156-194		
6	3	176	160-199		
6	4	181	164-204		

From Bray GA (editor): *Obesity in Perspective*. Fogarty International Center Series on Preventive Medicine, Vol.2, part I. D.H.E.W. Publication No. (NIH) 75-705. Washington, D.C. Department of Health, Education and Welfare, 1975.
[a] = Height without shoes   [b] = Weight without clothes.

V. INDICATIONS FOR PARENTERAL NUTRITION

Parenteral nutrition support is indicated in the presence of compromised nutritional status when adequate protein and calories cannot be provided by oral or other enteral routes. Depending on the degree of malnutrition, term of treatment and venous access, peripheral or central parenteral nutrition can be used. The following broad categories are considered indications for parenteral nutrition:

- Preoperative and postoperative support where malnutrition is a major problem (weight loss greater than 10%).

- When it is anticipated that a patient will not be able to ingest food for five days or longer, e.g., prolonged ileus, severe infection, or multiple diagnostic tests requiring the patient to be NPO.

- Premature neonatal patients with severe respiratory distress syndrome, necrotizing enterocolitis, malabsorption or other life threatening conditions.

- Neonatal congenital defects making enteral alimentation impossible: bowel atresia, gastroschisis, tracheoesophageal fistula.

- Patients with protracted emesis associated with pregnancy or chemotherapy.

- Patients with short bowel and malabsorption syndromes.

- Acutely ill patients with repeated aspiration.

- Conditions requiring complete bowel rest for a prolonged period of time: acute pancreatitis, enteric fistula, severe diarrhea.

- Patients with obstructing lesions of the gastrointestinal tract which prevent enteral alimentation: abdominal mass, small bowel obstruction or adhesions.

- Major trauma or burn patients when enteral alimentation is not possible, and/or with prolonged increased metabolic requirements.

- Patients with malignant disease which is being actively treated.

- Patients with active inflammatory bowel disease: ulcerative colitis, Crohn's disease.

- Patients who will not eat, such as patients with anorexia nervosa.

- Select patients with renal, cardiac or hepatic failure, as indicated by special circumstances and with expert advice.

- Comatose patients or patients with neurological conditions which interfere with eating.

VI. CENTRAL VENOUS CATHETER INSERTION GUIDELINES

A. General Principles

1. Insertion of a central line for PN is a surgical procedure and requires use of strict aseptic technique.

2. PN is **never** an emergency, and therefore, catheter insertion should be done under well controlled circumstances.

3. The patient's fears can be allayed and cooperation achieved through careful explanation of the procedure.

4. The infraclavicular approach is the preferred route.

5. The Trendelenburg position and a rolled sheet or towel along the vertebral column will allow for easier access to the subclavian vein.

6. The physician should wear a mask and gown, and all other personnel should wear masks during the entire procedure.

7. Preparation of the skin: shave hair, put on sterile gloves and cleanse site with a povidone-iodine solution.

8. A new pair of sterile gloves should be used to drape the area.

9. Important landmarks should be located; then local anesthetic is injected.

10. For a single lumen central venous catheter:

    a. The needle is inserted with the bevel pointing upward and pushed gently forward as the syringe is made to aspirate.

    b. Once the vein is entered and blood aspirated, the needle is immobilized with a hemostat.

    c. While the patient performs the Valsalva maneuver the syringe is removed, and the catheter is advanced through the needle until it seats in its hub.

    d. The catheter should never be pulled back through the needle; this can easily result in severing the catheter causing a catheter embolus.

    For a multilumen central venous catheter:

    a. All lumens must be flushed, filled, and connected to desired lines.

    b. A thin wall needle or introducer catheter may be used to introduce the guidewire into the vein.

    c. The tip of the guidewire should be inserted through the introducer needle or the catheter into the vein. If a "J" tip is used, slide the plastic tubing over the "J" to straighten it. Advance the guidewire to the desired depth. If using the "J" tip, a gentle rotating motion may be required.

d. The guidewire should be held in place and the introducer needle or catheter then removed. RETAIN FIRM CONTROL OF THE GUIDEWIRE AT ALL TIMES.

e. Enlargement of the cutaneous puncture site may be necessary with a dilator.

f. The tip of the multilumen catheter should be threaded over the guidewire. A slight twisting motion may be required to advance the catheter.

g. The catheter should be held in place at desired depth and the guidewire removed, leaving the catheter in place.

h. Attach syringe, aspirate until a free flow of venous blood is obtained.

11. Luer lock extension tubing that has been previously primed should then be attached securely to the catheter hub. Use only luer lock extension tubing.

12. The IV bottle should be lowered by an assistant to check for a prompt flashback of blood.

13. The needle guard for a single lumen catheter or a suture wing for the multilumen catheter is then fastened.

14. The needle guard assembly or the wing **lateral** must be sutured to the catheter on the anterior chest wall; this will promote catheter longevity and foster better catheter care.

15. The area should be dressed using the standard dressing kit and dressing protocol.

16. A chest x-ray must be obtained immediately to confirm proper catheter position, and to rule out technical complications, e.g., pneumothorax. The PN solution should not be started until x-ray confirmation of proper catheter position is obtained.

17. A note must be written in the chart, documenting the catheter insertion and confirming satisfactory catheter location by x-ray.

18. A guidewire may be used to exchange a catheter that requires replacement for mechanical reasons, but **not** for suspected or documented catheter sepsis due to increased risk of infecting the new catheter.

19. If a guidewire is used to exchange a catheter, a chest x-ray is mandatory to confirm proper catheter position and to rule out technical complications, e.g., pneumothorax.

B. Central Catheter Dressing Change

Sterility of the catheter-cutaneous junction and an occlusive dressing in place at all times are the keystones for catheter longevity. The following directions are for application of the first dressing only. Please refer to The Clinical Nursing Practice Manual for PN Patients for subsequent dressing changes which also provides guidelines for changing the extension tubing.

1. Set I.V. to a "keep open" rate.
2. Open sterile CVP dressing change kit, which contains all needed supplies.
3. Put on sterile gloves; set second pair aside.
4. Cleanse area with povidone-iodine swabsticks using clean-to-dirty technique x 3. When cleansing the multilumen catheter, the area from the catheter insertion site to approximately two inches along the catheter should be considered sterile.
5. Apply triple antibiotic ointment to insertion and suture sites with a cotton-tip applicator.
6. Cover the insertion site with a folded 4 x 4 gauze.
7. Place second folded 4 x 4 gauze to cover hub of catheter and first part of extension tubing for single lumen catheter or two inches of the exposed multilumen catheter.
8. Apply skin-prep around the 4 x 4 gauze; let air dry until smooth and shiny.
9. Apply tape over 4 x 4 gauze and beyond by approximately 3/4 inch. First, apply tape down the center of the dressing and then pinch tape around extension tubing for a single lumen catheter or around the catheter itself for a multilumen to achieve total occlusiveness. Then apply tape on both sides of the first piece of tape.
10. Bring a loop of extension tubing up to dressing and tape.
11. Adjust infusion to ordered rate once chest x-ray has been confirmed.
12. Write time, date, and initials on dressing. Central catheter dressing changes are to be done every 72 hours, if the dressing becomes loose or wet, if the patient complains of pain at the insertion site, or if the dressing is removed for any other reason.

VII. PERMANENT RIGHT ATRIAL CATHETERS (PRAC)

A. General

Permanent right atrial catheters (PRAC) may be used immediately, once proper placement is confirmed by chest x-ray. If the catheter must be used for multiple purposes and PN is to be infused, the recommended dextrose concentration is 10%. The use of the line for purposes other than PN should be avoided whenever possible. Special PRAC dressing change kits are available from Material Services Center.

B. Dressings

1. The protocol for the dressing change procedure is in The University of Michigan Hospitals Clinical Nursing Practice Manual which is located on each nursing unit. PEN Team Nurse Clinicians are available via paging for assistance.
2. Dressing changes with gauze should be done every 72 hours, or whenever the dressing becomes wet or loose, or needs to be changed for any other reason.

3. Transparent dressings are associated with increased microbial colonization under the dressing and increased catheter site infection, therefore they should not be used.

C. Care

1. For adults and pediatrics patients, irrigation of the PRAC with 5 mL of a heparinized saline solution (100 units/mL) should be done daily, after blood has been drawn or given, and after fluid or medication administration through the catheter. For neonates and newborn babies, irrigation should be done with 3 mL of a heparinized saline solution of 10 unit/mL. Irrigation should be done twice daily when the PRAC is not being used or irrigated as previously specified.

2. Irrigation should be done according to the protocol in The University of Michigan Hospitals Clinical Nursing Practice Manual.

3. Medical students may not draw blood from the PRAC unless certified to do so by a qualified house officer.

4. Padded hemostats or a catheter clamp specifically designed for PRAC should be kept at the bedside.

5. If resistance is encountered when the PRAC is irrigated, the physician should be notified immediately, as it may be necessary to use thrombolytic agents in order to prevent total catheter occlusion.

6. For additional information, review The Care of Permanent Right Atrial Catheter which is available from Educational Services for Nursing.

7. A senior house officer may be paged for assistance with catheter repair or a PEN Team member for those patients receiving PN support.

VIII. PARENTERAL NUTRITION SOLUTIONS FOR ADOLESCENT AND ADULT PATIENTS

A. Introduction

Prior to selecting a parenteral nutrition solution, caloric requirements should be determined. A detailed discussion of specific calculations of daily caloric needs is provided in Chapter IV, Section E. Protein, electrolyte, vitamin and trace element requirements are discussed later in this chapter.

There are five standard parenteral nutrition (PN) formulations available for adolescent and adult patients. Physicians are encouraged to prescribe standard formulations for their patients using the appropriate form designed for this purpose. When none of the standard PN formulations meet the needs of the patient, a detailed nonstandard PN order can then be prepared (See Section D, "Ordering Parenteral Nutrition Solutions.")

B. Components of Parenteral Nutrition Solutions

1. Dextrose

Hydrous dextrose has a caloric value of 3.4 kcal/g.

The final concentration of dextrose in most PN solutions for central administration is 25%. Patients on fluid restriction may receive up to 35% dextrose in the central PN solution. (Note: The Essential Amino Acid Formulation contains 43% dextrose, but in reduced total volume of 800 mL).

The final dextrose concentration in adult peripheral PN solutions is limited to 10% and the amino acid concentration to 2.5% due to the hyperosmolarity of the solution (880 mOsm/L). Hyperosmolarity, which can lead to vein irritation, can be reduced by the coadministration of fat emulsion (Appendix A).

The estimated glucose utilization rate by the liver ranges between 0.4 to 1.2 g/kg/hr. Glucose utilization is influenced by age and metabolic state. Decreased glucose utilization is seen with advancing age, diabetes mellitus, liver disease, sepsis, and stress (including major surgery and trauma). Physicians should not attempt to exceed the maximal rate of glucose utilization for their patients since hyperosmolar nonketotic hyperglycemia may result.

2. Protein

Protein has a caloric value of 4.0 kcal/g.

The recommended daily requirement for adult patients with relatively normal renal and liver function is 0.8 to 1.5 g/kg/day of protein.

The goal of nutritional support is to preserve the body's lean body mass (minimize protein breakdown) or replete protein stores that have been depleted secondary to disease (promote protein synthesis). To optimize nitrogen retention, sufficient energy substrates must be provided. The non-protein calorie-to-nitrogen ratio is used as an index to ensure maximum utilization of protein. The desired ratio ranges from 150 to 300 kcal from carbohydrate or fat sources to 1 gram of nitrogen (equivalent to 6.25 grams of protein). All standard mixed amino acid PN formulations meet this ratio when co-administered with fat emulsion.

There are three central amino acid solutions on The University of Michigan Hospitals Formulary. Their indications and use are described below.

a. Formulations for Central Vein Administration

Commonly, one liter of PN solution intended for central administration provides 42.5 grams of protein (Aminosyn® 8.5% — 500 mL) and a final dextrose concentration ranging from 25% to 35%.

1) Crystalline Amino Acids 8.5% (Aminosyn® 8.5% — Abbott), 500 mL. This solution provides essential and nonessential amino acids as follows:

Essential Amino Acids	(mg/100 mL)	Non-essential Amino Acids	(mg/100 mL)
L-Isoleucine	620	L-Alanine	1100
L-Leucine	810	L-Arginine	850
L-Lysine Acetate	624	L-Histidine	260
L-Methionine	340	L-Proline	750
L-Phenylalanine	380	L-Serine	370
L-Threonine	460	L-Tyrosine	44
L-Tryptophan	150	Glycine	1100
L-Valine	680	(Aminoacetic Acid,USP)	

500 mL of Aminosyn® 8.5% provides 42.5 grams of protein equivalent to 6.7 grams of nitrogen. Electrolyte content includes 2.7 mEq of potassium, 45 mEq of acetate, and 17.5 mEq of chloride.

2) Crystalline Amino Acids 10% (Aminosyn® 10% — Abbott), 500 mL. This solution provides essential and nonessential amino acids as follows:

Essential Amino Acids	(mg/100 mL)	Non-essential Amino Acids	(mg/100 mL)
L-Isoleucine	720	L-Alanine	1280
L-Leucine	940	L-Arginine	980
L-Lysine Acetate	720	L-Histidine	300
L-Methionine	400	L-Proline	860
L-Phenylalanine	440	L-Serine	420
L-Threonine	520	L-Tyrosine	44
L-Tryptophan	160	Glycine	1280
L-Valine	800	(Aminoacetic Acid,USP)	

500 mL of Aminosyn® 10% provides 50 grams of protein equivalent to 7.9 grams of nitrogen. Electrolyte content includes 2.7 mEq of potassium, 74 mEq of acetate. This solution has an osmolarity of 1000 mOsm/L.

3) Essential Amino Acid Solution 5.2% (Aminosyn-RF® 5.2% — Abbott), 300 mL. Aminosyn-RF® 5.2% provides histidine, a nonessential amino acid thought to be essential in the uremic patient, and arginine, in addition to the eight essential amino acids. The amino acid profile is as follows:

Essential Amino Acids	(mg/100 mL)	Non-essential Amino Acids	(mg/100 mL)
L-Isoleucine	462	L-Arginine	600
L-Leucine	726	L-Histidine	429
L-Lysine Acetate	535		
L-Methionine	726		
L-Phenylalanine	726		
L-Threonine	330		
L-Tryptophan	165		
L-Valine	528		

300 mL of Aminosyn-RF® 5.2% provides 15.7 grams of protein equivalent to 2.4 grams of nitrogen. Electrolyte content includes 1.5 mEq of potassium and 31.5 mEq of acetate. This solution has an osmolarity of 475 mOsm/L.

b. Formulations for Peripheral Vein Administration

One liter of PN solution for peripheral administration provides 25 grams of protein and a final dextrose concentration of 10%.

1) Crystalline Amino Acid Solution 5% (Aminosyn® 5% — Abbott), 500 ml. This solution provides essential and nonessential amino acids as follows:

Essential Amino Acids	(mg/100 ml)	Non-essential Amino Acids	(mg/100 ml)
L-Isoleucine	360	L-Alanine	640
L-Leucine	470	L-Arginine	490
L-Lysine Acetate	360	L-Histidine	150
L-Methionine	200	L-Proline	430
L-Phenylalanine	220	L-Serine	210
L-Threonine	260	L-Tyrosine	44
L-Tryptophan	80	Glycine	640
L-Valine	400	(Aminoacetic Acid,USP)	

500 ml of Aminosyn® 5% provides 25 grams of protein equivalent to 3.9 grams of nitrogen. Electrolyte content includes 2.7 mEq of potassium and 43 mEq of acetate. This solution has an osmolarity of 500 mOsm/L.

c. Renal Failure Regimens

In patients with renal failure, modified nutritional support regimens with protein restriction have been used to reduce uremic symptoms. Whether patients clinically benefit from special essential amino acid formulations over low-dose standard amino acid formulations remains controversial. Optimal nutritional support in patients with acute renal failure is often times difficult to achieve due to fluid limitations, electrolyte imbalances, and rising BUN/Cr. Dextrose can be administered in a final concentration of 35% to limit the fluid load. Hemofiltration (Continuous Arteriovenous Hemofiltration, Slow Continuous Ultrafiltration) and dialysis (Hemodialysis, Continuous Arteriovenous Hemofiltration-Dialysis) procedures are used to provide a means for nitrogenous waste, electrolyte and fluid elimination allowing physicians to optimize nutritional support in the renal failure patient. Glucose tolerance, adequate excretion of nitrogenous wastes and fluid loads must all be carefully monitored to avoid further insult to renal function.

1) Non-standard formulation: (2.5% mixed nonessential and essential amino acids, 35% dextrose in one liter). This formulation provides reduced protein and increased calories in a minimal volume of fluid. Electrolyte content must be specified. This allows the physician flexibility in adjusting the electrolyte content (i.e., potassium, phosphate, magnesium) of the PN solution based on the patient's renal status. Non-standard order forms (H-2060401) should be used to order this parenteral nutrition solution.

2) Essential Amino Acid formulation: (Aminosyn-RF® 5.2%, 300 ml, mixed with 70% dextrose, 500 ml, for a final dextrose concentration of 43% in a total volume 800 ml). This provides a low protein and high calorie formulation for patients where it is desirable to restrict fluid and protein.

Clinical judgment is required in selecting nutritional support for renal failure patients, and adjustments in nutritional support on a daily basis may be necessary.

d. Hepatic Failure Regimen

Patients suffering from hepatic dysfunction generally should not receive more than a total daily protein load of 40-50 grams from standard amino acid solutions in order to prevent serum amino acid imbalances, metabolic alkalosis, pre-renal azotemia, and hyperammonemia. A standard PN formulation with mixed amino acids diluted to 2.5% can be ordered if the prescriber is concerned with encephalopathy. Amino acid administration should be stopped if the patient exhibits stupor and coma.

3. Electrolytes

a. Electrolyte Requirements

It is recommended that all adult patients be supplemented with electrolytes in each bottle in the ranges listed below on a daily basis unless contraindicated:

Calcium	10 - 15	mEq/day (5 mEq/L)
Magnesium	8 - 24	mEq/day (5-8 mEq/L)
Potassium*	90 - 240	mEq/day (20-50 mEq/L)
Sodium	60 - 150	mEq/day (20-50 mEq/L)
Acetate*	80 - 120	mEq/day (30-50 mEq/L)
Chloride*	60 - 150	mEq/day (20-50 mEq/L)
Phosphorus	30 - 50	mM/day (10-15 mM/L)

* Amino acid solution 5% (Aminosyn® 5% - 500 mL) provides 43 mEq acetate and 2.7 mEq potassium.
Amino acid solution 8.5% (Aminosyn® 8.5% - 500 mL) provides 45 mEq acetate, 17.5 mEq chloride, and 2.7 mEq potassium.
Amino acid solution 10% (Aminosyn® 10% - 500 mL) provides 74 mEq acetate and 2.7 mEq potassium.
Essential amino acid solution 5.2% (Aminosyn® -RF 5.2% - 300 mL) provides 31.5 mEq acetate and 1.5 mEq potassium.

b. Single Electrolyte Formulations

Single electrolyte formulations are available for physicians to provide individual electrolytes to patients with high maintenance requirements or replacement needs. The following eight electrolyte salts are available:

Calcium	(Gluconate)	0.5 mEq/mL
Magnesium	(Sulfate)	4.0 mEq/mL
Potassium	(Chloride)	2.0 mEq/mL
	(Acetate)	2.0 mEq/mL
Sodium	(Chloride)	4.0 mEq/mL
	(Acetate)	2.0 mEq/mL
Phosphate*	(Potassium)	3.0 mM/mL
	(Sodium)	3.0 mM/mL

*When ordered as potassium phosphate, each prescribed millimole of phosphorus will contribute 1.47 mEq of potassium. One millimole of sodium phosphate will contribute 1.3 mEq of sodium.

4. Vitamins

   a. Multivitamin Infusion-12 (M.V.C. 9+3® - Lyphomed): 10 mL Mix-O-Vial®

   This is a vitamin preparation containing a combination of fat and water soluble vitamins. This preparation meets the AMA Guidelines for Vitamin Therapy except for Vitamin K. One 10 ml vial contains the following vitamins:

Ascorbic Acid	100.0	mg
Vitamin A	3,300.0	IU
Vitamin D	200.0	IU
Thiamine HCl (B_1)	3.0	mg
Riboflavin (B_2)	3.6	mg
Pyridoxine HCl (B_6)	4.0	mg
Niacinamide	40.0	mg
Pantothenic Acid	15.0	mg
Vitamin E	10.0	IU
Biotin	60	mcg
Folic Acid	400	mcg
Cyanocobalamin (B_{12})	5	mcg

When a physician prescribes a standard PN formulation, the above vitamin formulation will be added by the Pharmacy. When the patient is on a non-standardized solution, it is the physician's responsibility to indicate whether or not the multivitamins should be added to the PN solution. The PEN Team recommends 10 ml to be administered every day.

   b. Phytonadione - Vitamin K_1 (AquaMephyton® - MSD)

When a physician prescribes a standard PN formulation, Vitamin K_1 5 mg will be added by the Pharmacy to the parenteral nutrition every Monday on a weekly basis. When multivitamins are ordered on a Monday in a non-standard solution, Vitamin K_1 5 mg will be added by the Pharmacy. It is the physician's responsibility to request the deletion of the Vitamin K_1 from the Monday PN order for those patients that should not receive Vitamin K_1.

5. Trace Elements

   a. Multi-Trace Element Formulation for Adults (MTE-5® Concentrate - Lyphomed). Each 1 mL of this formulation contains the following:

Zinc	(as sulfate)	5.0	mg
Copper	(as sulfate)	1.0	mg
Manganese	(as sulfate)	0.5	mg
Chromium	(as chloride)	0.010	mg
Selenium	(as selenious acid)	0.060	mg

One ml of the Multi-Trace Element Formulation should be administered in the PN solution every day. When standard PN formulations are ordered, trace elements are added automatically. Additional individual trace elements can be provided in the PN solution for suspected or diagnosed single trace element deficiencies. This trace element formulation meets the requirement of the stable adult for zinc and other trace elements.

However, the AMA Nutrition Advisory Group (JPEN, 3:263, 1979) suggests an additional 2 mg of zinc daily for adults in acute catabolic states. The following additional zinc should be provided in stable adults with intestinal losses:

17 mg/l of stool or ileostomy output

The Nutrition Advisory Group stresses, however, that frequent monitoring of blood levels in these patients is essential to provide proper dosage.

b. Single Trace Element Formulations

Single trace element formulations are available for physicians to provide individual trace metals to patients with high metabolic or replacement needs, and to treat a suspected or diagnosed trace element deficiency. The following six formulations are available:

Chromium	(as chloride)	0.004 mg/mL
Copper	(as chloride)	0.4 mg/mL
Manganese	(as sulfate)	0.1 mg/mL
Molybdenum	(as ammonium)	0.025 mg/mL
Selenium	(as selenious acid)	0.04 mg/mL
Zinc	(as chloride)	1.0 mg/mL

6. Other Additives to the Parenteral Nutrition Solutions

a. Heparin: Heparin sodium should be provided in the PN solution in a concentration of 1 unit/mL. Thus, each liter of PN will contain 1000 units of heparin. This is to reduce the formation of a fibrin sheath around the catheter and possibly to reduce the phlebitis in patients receiving peripherally infused PN solutions.

b. Iron dextran (Imferon® — Fisons Corp): A test dose must be given before addition to PN solutions. Twenty five milligrams of iron dextron in 50 to 100 mL of a dextrose 5%-in-water or 0.9% Sodium Chloride should be administered over at least 15 minutes. Patients should be observed for any hypersensitivity reaction during administration. For iron deficiency not due to blood loss, the total replacement dosage (in mg of elemental iron) to be administered may be calculated as follows:

$$\text{mg Iron} = 0.66 \times BW \times \left[100 - \frac{\text{Hgb}(100)}{14.8} \right]$$

BW = body weight in kg
Hgb = hemoglobin in g%

Up to 100 mg of iron dextran can be added to each 24 hr supply of PN solution until the total replacement dosage has been administered. Iron dextran should not be added to the adult patient's solution routinely or for prophylaxis.

c. Regular Human Insulin: Exogenous regular human insulin may be added to the PN solution when glucose intolerance and glycosuria persist despite an initial slow infusion rate of the PN solution. Blood glucose levels should not be allowed to persist at levels above 200 mg/dl. Because some insulin will absorb to the TPN container and IV tubing, at least 10 units of insulin should be added per liter of PN solution.

d. Hydrochloric Acid: Patients on nasogastric suction or with high-output enterocutaneous fistula or on intensive IV diuretic therapy are prone to metabolic alkalosis because of the high chloride and potassium losses. **PN solutions should not be used as a replacement solution for these losses.** Rather replacement should be volume-for-volume with an electrolyte solution which closely approximates the electrolyte content of the fluid loss. Patients with documented severe metabolic alkalosis and in whom sodium and potassium restriction is necessary may have hydrochloric acid (up to 100 mEq/liter) added to the central parenteral nutrition solution. Administration of HCL requires frequent monitoring of blood pH and serum electrolytes, as acidosis may develop quickly. Hydrochloric acid should never be administered routinely, or for treatment of mild metabolic alkalosis. Proper fluid and electrolyte replacement is always the appropriate therapy.

7. Fat

Fat has a caloric value of 9 kcal/g.

The indications for the use of fat emulsion in patients supported by PN are to treat or prevent essential fatty acid deficiency and to provide a concentrated calorie source. Patients may develop biochemical evidence of essential fatty acid deficiency within a week while on PN. The clinical signs of the deficiency, however may take a month or more to manifest. When used to prevent essential fatty acid deficiency, fat should constitute at least 4% of the daily caloric intake of the patient as linoleic acid. Minimum essential fatty acid requirements may be satisfied by administering 500 mL of fat emulsion, 10%, twice weekly or 500 mL of fat emulsion, 20%, weekly. The maximum recommended dose of fat for treating essential fatty acid deficiency, and when used as a caloric source, is 3 g/kg/day for adults. Exceeding this dosage guideline may precipitate a fat overload syndrome. Fat emulsion supplementation should not constitute more than 60% of the daily caloric intake. It should be noted that 500 mL of the fat emulsion 10% has a total caloric value of 550 kcal. This is due to the caloric contribution by the glycerol and the egg phosphatide, in addition to the fat content in the emulsion (50 g). On the other hand, 500 mL of fat emulsion 20% has a caloric value of 1000 kcal.

Fat emulsion can be administered concomitantly with PN solutions. It can be infused peripherally or centrally without untoward effect. It is always advisable, however to infuse fat peripherally whenever the peripheral parenteral nutrition formulation is prescribed (2.5% amino acids and 10% dextrose) in order to reduce the overall osmolarity of the solution. A test dose should be administered at a rate of 1.0 mL/minute for the first 15 minutes. If no adverse effects are observed during this initial infusion, the rate can then be increased. Fat emulsion should never be administered through a 0.22 micron filter nor should electrolytes or other additives be added to it. Due to the establishment of generic equivalency between Intralipid® (soybean fat emulsion), and Liposyn® II (soybean/safflower oil fat emulsion), the University of Michigan Hospitals may stock either brand name product.

a. Soybean Oil Fat Emulsion 10% (Intralipid® 10% Kabivitrum), 500 mL. This emulsion contains the following:

Soybean Oil	10.0 %
Egg Phospholipids	1.2 %
Glycerin	2.25%
Water for Injection q.s.	500.0 mL

The soybean oil is a mixture of neutral triglycerides of predominantly unsaturated fatty acids. The fatty acids forming the major components of the emulsion are:

Linoleic Acid	50%
Oleic Acid	26%
Palmitic Acid	10%
Linolenic Acid	9%

A 500 mL bottle provides 50 grams of fat, has an osmolarity of 260 mOsm/L, and provides a total of 550 kcal (1.1 kcal/mL).

b. Soybean Oil Fat Emulsion 20% (Intralipid® 20%, Kabivitrum)

The percent composition of Soybean Oil Fat Emulsion 20% is as that of 10% listed under (a) above. A 500 mL bottle provides 100 grams of fat, has an osmolarity of 268 mOsm/L, and provides a total of 1000 kcal (2.0 kcal/mL).

c. Soybean/Safflower Oil Fat Emulsion 10% (Liposyn® II 10% - Abbott), 500 mL. This emulsion contains the following:

Soybean Oil	5.0%
Safflower Oil	5.0%
Egg Phosphatides	up to 1.2%
Glycerin	2.5%
Water for Injection q.s.	500.0mL

The soybean/safflower oil is a mixture of neutral triglycerides of predominantly unsaturated fatty acids. The fatty acids forming the major component of the emulsion are:

Linoleic Acid	65.8%
Oleic Acid	17.7%
Palmitic Acid	8.8%
Stearic Acid	3.4%
Linolenic Acid	4.2%

A 500 mL bottle provides 50 grams of fat, has an osmolarity of 276 mOsm/L and provides a total of 550 kcal.

d. Soybean/Safflower Oil Fat Emulsion 20% (Liposyn® II 20% - Abbott) The percent composition of Soybean/Safflower Oil Fat Emulsion 20% is as that of 10% listed under (c) above. A 500 mL bottle provides 100 grams of fat, has an osmolarity of 258 mOsm/L, and provides a total of 1000 kcal.

e. Both 10% and 20% fat emulsion contain between 4.3 and 8.0 mM bound phosphate per 500 mL bottle.

C. Stability and Compatibilities

1. Expiration Time

   Each parenteral nutrition solution dispensed from the Pharmacy will be given a 2:00 p.m. (or 10:00 a.m. in Mott) expiration time. The expiration date will be 24 hours from the scheduled administration time. No parenteral nutrition solution may be administered beyond the expiration date and time specified on the label.

   Please return unused PN bottles to the
   Pharmacy, so that the patient is credited.

2. Refrigeration

   Refrigeration is not required as long as the expiration date printed on each parenteral nutrition solution bottle is strictly observed. However, all bottles should be stored in a dark, cool place.

3. Additives

   a. Electrolyte Limits

   Electrolytes in the concentrations listed are compatible when added to 1000 mL of parenteral nutrition solution. Ordering electrolytes in concentrations exceeding the recommended range may result in precipitation or lack of biological availability of these electrolytes as prescribed.

Calcium*	up to 30 mEq* (dependent on phosphate content)
Magnesium	up to 20 mEq
Potassium	up to 80 mEq
Sodium	up to 155 mEq
Acetate	Wide Range
Chloride	Wide Range
Phosphorus*	up to 30 mM* (dependent on calcium content)

   *Calcium-phosphorus compatibility can be determined by the following equation:

   Calcium (mEq) + phosphorus (mM) ≤ "30" (per 1000 mL)

   A sum greater than 30 indicates a high potential for precipitation to occur either instantly or at a later time during solution administration.

   b. Drugs

   Compatibility of drugs in parenteral solutions should not be assumed when incompatibility data are lacking. No drug can be added to any protein and dextrose parenteral nutrition solution other than vitamins recommended for intravenous infusion, electrolytes, trace elements, heparin, insulin, hydrochloric acid, iron dextran, cimetidine and ranitidine.

   The following list presents medications compatible with parenteral nutrition solutions only (e.g., amino acids, dextrose, electrolytes, trace elements and vitamins) when administered via a piggyback system into the parenteral nutrition line. Compatibility data on fat emulsions is limited and consists of physical compatibility only; therefore, fat emulsion infusions must be interrupted to run in all medications. Note that common parenteral nutrition ingredients (e.g., electrolytes, multivitamins, trace elements) and common intravenous fluids (dextrose 5%, saline solutions and lactated ringer's) are considered compatible when administered via piggyback systems. Fat emulsion may be co-administered with these medication-free solutions.

Medications Physically and Chemically Compatible with UMMC Parenteral Nutrition Solutions When Administered via a Piggyback System[1,2]

Aminophylline[3]	Hydrochloric Acid
Ampicillin[3]	Imipenim-Cilastin
Carbenicillin	Insulin (regular)
Cefazolin	Kanamycin
Cefotaxime	Meperidine
Ceftazidine	Methicillin
Ceftriaxone	Metoclopramide
Chloramphenicol	Methotrexate
Cimetidine[4,5]	Mezlocillin
Clindamycin	Morphine[3]
Cyclophosphamide	Nitroglycerine
Cytarabine	Penicillin G
Digoxin	Piperacillin
Dobutamine	Polymyxin B
Famotidine[4,5]	Ranitidine[4,5]
Fluorouracil	Thiamine[5]
Folic Acid[5]	Ticarcillin
Gentamicin	Tobramycin
Heparin	Vancomycin HCL

Notes: 1. Mixing via piggyback systems above filter only. Data do not support direct mixing of medication with PN solutions in an in-line drip chamber (e.g., buretrol).
2. Low dextrose peripheral formulations (Dextrose 10%) must be utilized when co-administering medications with PN solutions.
3. Concentration or dose dependent, maximum concentration of piggyback fluid:

Aminophylline	3 mg/mL
Ampicillin	10 mg/mL
Morphine	2 mg/mL

4. Recommended intravenous doses:

Cimetidine (300 mg vial)	900 – 1200 mg/day normal renal function.
	600 – 900 mg/day renal failure.
Rantidine (50 mg vial)	150 – 200 mg/day normal renal function.
	50 – 75 mg/day renal failure.
Famotidine (20 mg vial)	20 – 40 mg/day normal renal function.
	10 – 20 mg/day renal failure.

5. May be directly admixed with TPN solution. Fat emulsion can be co-administered.

For further compatibility information call the PEN Team at 936-8231 or the Drug Information Service at 936-8200.

D. Ordering Parenteral Nutrition Solutions

Parenteral nutrition solutions for adults can be ordered on either of two order and administration forms, depending on whether the solutions being ordered are standard or non-standard formulations. The PEN Team recommends that physicians order standard PN formulations for their patients, unless this is clinically contraindicated. Listed below is a description of the procedure to be followed in ordering standard and non-standard PN formulations.

1. Standard PN Formulations

   Orders for standard PN solutions should be written on the form:

   DAILY PARENTERAL NUTRITION (PN) ORDER AND ADMINISTRATION FORM FOR STANDARD FORMULATION FOR ADOLESCENT AND ADULT PATIENTS #H-2060413 (Appendix B)

   It is anticipated that the five standard formulations listed on this form will meet the clinical and nutritional needs of the majority of adult patients.

   The following are guidelines for filling out this form:

   a. Patient's name and location should be plated.

   b. The prescriber should choose the standard formulation which most closely meets the needs of the patient by recording the PN solution sequence number in the box corresponding to the desired solution. The PN sequence number is a serial number given to each PN solution order by the prescriber which dictates the appropriate administration sequence. PN sequence numbers should be continuous as long as the patient is on PN. The detailed content of each of the standard formulations is printed on the back of the order form and in this publication.

   c. Should there be clinical need to increase supplementation of any ingredient, this can be requested in the space provided for this purpose. The PN sequence number of the solution that needs the alteration, followed by the order should be specified. An increased concentration of different ingredients can be requested in any PN solution, provided these requests conform to the maximum compatibility limits stated under the section on Instability and Incompatibilities.

   d. The flow rate per hour should be specified in the corresponding box. The volume of PN solution should be ordered with consistent flow rates over a 24 hour period.

   e. Fat emulsion should be ordered on the PN order form designating the desired percent emulsion and the flow rate.

   f. The prescriber should specify the date when the PN solution is to be administered along with his/her signature, pager number and date written.

   g. Individual Standard PN Formulations

      The standard parenteral nutrition formulations that can be ordered for adolescent and adult patients are listed on the next page:

Mixed Amino Acid Formulation

Amino Acids (4.25%)	42.5	g	**Approximate Volume**
Dextrose (25%)	250	g	1050 mL
Calcium	4.5	mEq	**Approximate Osmolarity**
Magnesium	5	mEq	1825 mOsm/L
Potassium	40	mEq	
Sodium	35	mEq	**Total Caloric Value**
Acetate	74.5	mEq	1020 kcal
Chloride	52.5	mEq	(approx. 1 kcal/mL)
Phosphorus	12	mM	
Heparin Sodium	1000	units	**Nitrogen Content**
*Multivitamins with Biotin,			6.7 g
B$_{12}$ and Folic Acid	10	mL	
*Trace Elements	1	mL	**Non-Protein Calorie/g Nitrogen**
**Vitamin K$_1$	5	mg	127:1

Mixed Amino Acid Formulation: Low Potassium and Added Sodium

Amino Acids (4.25%)	42.5	g	**Approximate Volume**
Dextrose (25%)	250	g	1050 mL
Calcium	4.5	mEq	**Approximate Osmolarity**
Magnesium	5	mEq	1825 mOsm/L
Potassium	23	mEq	
Sodium	51	mEq	**Total Caloric Value**
Acetate	74.5	mEq	1020 kcal
Chloride	52.5	mEq	(approx. 1 kcal/mL)
Phosphorus	12	mM	
(approx. 1 kcal/mL)			
Heparin Sodium	1000	units	**Nitrogen Content**
*Multivitamins with Biotin,			6.7 g
B$_{12}$ and Folic Acid	10	mL	
*Trace Elements	1	mL	**Non-Protein Calorie/g Nitrogen**
**Vitamin K$_1$	5	mg	127:1

Mixed Amino Acid Cardiac Formulation (No Sodium Added)

Amino Acids (4.25%)	42.5	g	**Approximate Volume**
Dextrose (35%)	350	g	1050 mL
Calcium	4.5	mEq	
Magnesium	8	mEq	**Approximate Osmolarity**
Potassium	40	mEq	2325 mOsm/L
Acetate	45	mEq	
Chloride	37.5	mEq	**Total Caloric Value**
Gluconate	4.5	mEq	1360 kcal
Sulfate	8	mEq	(approx. 1.4 kcal/mL)
Phosphorus	12	mM	
Heparin Sodium	1000	units	**Nitrogen Content**
*Multivitamins with Biotin,			6.7 g
B$_{12}$ and Folic Acid	10	mL	
*Trace Elements	1	mL	**Non-Protein Calorie/g Nitrogen**
**Vitamin K$_1$	5	mg	178:1

Essential Amino Acid Formulation

Essential Amino Acids (2%)	15.7	g	**Approximate Volume**
Dextrose (43%)	350	g	800 mL
Potassium	1.6	mEq	**Approximate Osmolarity**
Acetate	31.5	mEq	1935 mOsm/L
Heparin Sodium	1000	units	**Total Caloric Value**
*Multivitamins with Biotin,			1253 kcal
B$_{12}$ and Folic Acid	10	mL	(approx. 1.66 kcal/mL)
			Nitrogen Content
			2.5 g
**Vitamin K$_1$	5	mg	**Non-Protein Calorie/g Nitrogen**
			476:1

Mixed Amino Acid Peripheral Formulation

Amino Acids (2.5%)	25	g	**Approximate Volume**
Dextrose (10%)	100	g	1050 mL
Calcium	4.5	mEq	
Magnesium	5	mEq	**Approximate Osmolarity**
Potassium	23	mEq	880 mOsm/L
Sodium	47	mEq	
Acetate	82	mEq	**Total Caloric Value**
Chloride	35	mEq	440 kcal
Phosphorus	9	mM	(approx. 0.43 kcal/mL)
Heparin Sodium	1000	units	
*Multivitamins with Biotin,			**Nitrogen Content**
B$_{12}$ and Folic Acid	10	mL	4.0 g
*Trace Elements	1	mL	**Non-Protein Calorie/g Nitrogen**
**Vitamin K$_1$	5	mg	85:1

Note: Administration of 500 mL fat emulsion 10% with this solution results in a 222:1 non-protein calorie/g nitrogen. Due to the high osmolarity of this peripheral solution, it should be infused concurrently with fat emulsion. Also see notes on following page.

* Multivitamins and trace elements will be added daily to the parenteral nutrition solution.

** Vitamin K$_1$ will be added weekly (Monday) to the parenteral nutrition solution.

Vitamins, trace elements and heparin will be added automatically to all standard formulations as follows:

1) Multivitamin Infusion, 10 mL, will be added each day to the PN solution. Vitamin K_1, 5 mg, will also be added on a weekly basis (Monday).

For patients on anticoagulation therapy, it is the physician's responsibility to request the deletion of Vitamin K, from the parenteral nutrition solution, when deemed appropriate.

2) Multi-Trace Element Formulation for Adults, 1 mL, will be added to each day's order of standard PN formulations, except to the Essential Amino Acid Formulations.

3) Heparin Sodium, 1000 units, will be added daily to every liter of standard PN solution.

2. Non-Standard PN Formulations

Orders for non-standard PN solutions should be written on the form:

DAILY PARENTERAL NUTRITION (PN) ORDER AND ADMINISTRATION FORM FOR ADOLESCENT AND ADULT PATIENTS #H-2060401 (Appendix C)

This form should be used when none of the standard formulations meet the patient's requirements, or when a deletion of any ingredient from a standard formulation is indicated.

The following are guidelines for filling out this form:

a. Patient's name and location should be plated.

b. The total volume of PN solution should be specified by writing the PN sequence number in each of the PN sequence number boxes. The PN solution is ordered on a per liter basis with each liter being assigned a sequence number. The final dextrose and amino acid concentrations must also be specified in the corresponding spaces. Table 6 provides a guideline for amino acid and dextrose concentrations in non-standard PN formulations.

c. The flow rate per hour should be specified in the corresponding box. The volume of PN solution should be ordered with consistent flow rates over a 24 hour period.

d. Fat emulsion should be ordered on a PN order form designating the desired percent emulsion and the flow rate.

e. The prescriber should specify the date when the ordered PN solution is to be administered along with his/her signature, pager number and date written.

TABLE 6

GUIDELINES FOR AMINO ACID AND DEXTROSE CONCENTRATIONS IN NON-STANDARD PN SOLUTIONS

Type of Patient	Total Volume of TPN Solution to be Ordered Per Bottle	Final Concentration of Crystalline Amino Acid Solution	Final Concentration of Essential Amino Acid Solution	Final Concentration of Dextrose Solution
Normal liver and renal function	1000 mL	4.25%	—	25% (central infusion)
Chronic or acute renal failure	a) 800 mL b) 1000 mL	— 2.5 %	2.0% —	43% (central infusion) 35% (central infusion)
Liver dysfunction	1000 mL	2.5 %	—	25% (central infusion)
Cardiac patient with fluid restriction	1000 mL	4.25%	—	35% (central infusion)
Peripheral supplementation for patients with normal renal and liver function	1000 mL	2.5 %	—	10% (peripheral infusion)

f. Additives are ordered per liter of PN. Please see the section on General Requirements for Parenteral Nutrition in this chapter for recommended daily dosages.

If the clinical status of the patient necessitates the alteration of the PN solution after it has been compounded, the prescribing physician should write a new order and have the previous PN solution returned to the pharmacy. If the solution is still in the Pharmacy, the appropriate changes will be made as soon as the new order form is received. In either case, the alteration or recompounding of any solution will be made by the Pharmacy upon receipt of the physician's order. In the event that any PN solution has to be compounded again due to precipitation or breakage, dextrose solution 10% should be hung, and the prescriber notified if the administration of the latter is expected to last longer than one hour.

E. Daily Orders and Delivery

A separate PN order and administration form should be filled out each day by the physician and sent to the Pharmacy by 9:00 p.m. of the evening prior to solution administration. Orders received after 9:00 p.m. will be processed as soon as the compounding schedule allows. Late orders will not be given priority over orders received on time or new orders. PN solutions should be ordered to last from 2:00 p.m. of one day until 2:00 p.m. of the next day. Solutions ordered to last beyond a 24-hour period will automatically be cancelled by the Pharmacy unless the nurse or prescriber communicates with the Pharmacy verifying the order, such as when anticipating an increase in the flow rate. When the Pharmacy cancels any PN solution, a note of the cancellation will be sent with the same day's supply of PN solution.

All PN solutions ordered by 9:00 p.m. of the evening prior to administration will be delivered by 1:00 p.m. of the next day. Please inform the Pharmacy (936-8244) whenever the patient's parenteral nutrition support is discontinued. This is to avoid waste and charging the patients for therapy they are not expected to receive.

F. Administration and Discontinuation of Parenteral Nutrition Solutions

The infusion of hyperosmolar solutions without due consideration can lead to hyperglycemia and water depletion. Glucose intolerance can be seen in patients with latent or overt diabetes mellitus, stress, sepsis, or shock. Infusion rates for hypertonic dextrose solutions must be slow initially, and increased while monitoring urine and blood glucose. The infusion rate can be increased as the ability to tolerate the glucose increases. The following are guidelines for starting patients on PN:

1. One liter of central PN solution should be ordered for the first 24 hours to avoid wastage and hyperglycemic complications. Because of the reduced dextrose concentration in the peripheral solution, two liters of PN solution may be ordered on day one of infusion.
2. For patients receiving PN solution with 25% dextrose, start at 40 mL/hr/day and increase the rate by 40 mL/hr/day until the infusion rate desired is achieved.
3. For patients receiving PN solution with 35-43% dextrose, start at 30 mL/hr/day and increase the rate by 20 mL/hr/day until the infusion rate desired is achieved.

Whenever the hypertonic dextrose infusion is stopped suddenly, rebound hypoglycemia can occur. The infusion must, therefore, never be interrupted for infusion of other fluids. If surgery is contemplated during total parenteral nutrition support, the infusion rate should be reduced by one half, or the PN solution should be replaced with 10% dextrose solution immediately before, during, and shortly after surgery.

When the PN infusion is to be discontinued, this should be done either by gradually decreasing the rate of infusion over a few days, by giving isotonic glucose for at least six hours after stopping the hypertonic glucose, or by ensuring adequate caloric intake by means of the GI tract before discontinuing the PN solution.

It is recommended that the PN solution be discontinued by reversing the manner in which it was started, as described above.

Nurses are to record administration of PN solutions on the IV administration record or 24 hour flow sheet which becomes a permanent part of the patient's record.

G. Transition Period

Few patients remain on parenteral nutrition permanently. It is important, therefore, that transition from parenteral to enteral support be initiated before parenteral support is discontinued.

For patients transitioning to P.O. support, calorie counts ordered during this period allow the clinician to quantitate intake and choose the most advantageous way to reduce parenteral nutrition. When ordered, calorie counts begin the next day and continue for three days. Daily results are posted at the patient's door. The three day total, when complete, is recorded in the patient's chart. Guidelines for transitional feedings in patients with nasoenteric or tube enterostomies are detailed in Chapter XIII, Section F.

IX. ADMINISTRATION POLICIES AND TECHNIQUES

A. General

Hypertonic PN solution should not be infused before satisfactory catheter position has been confirmed by X-ray. The PN catheter and administration set are the patient's life line, and their integrity should not be violated. The PN line should not be used for central venous pressure readings (CVP's), to administer blood products, for "piggyback" medications, for blood drawing, or for fluids for hydration, unless absolutely necessary. Such violations are associated with a higher incidence of mechanical line failure and septic episodes.

B. Dressings

1. The protocol for the dressing change procedure is in The Clinical Nursing Practice Manual which is located on each nursing unit. PEN nurse clinicians are always available via paging for assistance. The protocol is also located in the CVC dressing change kit.
2. Dressing changes are done every 72 hours for a subclavian line, or whenever the dressing is wet or loose.
3. Dressing changes for a jugular line are done every 24 to 48 hours due to the difficulty of maintaining an occlusive dressing for greater than 24 to 48 hours.
4. Transparent dressings are associated with increased microbial colonization under the dressing and increased catheter site infection, therefore they shall not be used. The only exception would be in the case of a patient with a tracheostomy that is draining copious secretions near a catheter exit site.

5. Luer lock extension tubing that is connected to the central catheter underneath the dressing should be changed only when the dressing is changed, i.e., every 72 hours.

6. If the patient is going to the O.R. with a line that is being used for PN, identify the PN line with a label marked PN so Anesthesia and Recovery Room personnel will be aware of its purpose and restrict its use except for emergency situations.

C. Catheters

1. Currently there are three types of percutaneous catheters available: single lumen, bi or double lumen and a triple lumen. The number of lumens selected should be based on the patient's clinical condition. Extra lumens which will not be used should be avoided.

2. The middle lumen of the triple lumen, and the proximal lumen of the double lumen, should be designated the TPN lumen and should be treated as such for the duration of insertion.

3. If a lumen of the triple lumen is no longer needed, it may be maintained as a heparin lock following the same procedure used for heparinizing the permanent right atrial catheter once daily.

4. When two lumens of the triple lumen catheter are no longer needed, it should be replaced with a single lumen catheter.

5. The single lumen central catheter currently used is eight-inches in length. Noting the total length exposed is important, because occasionally the catheter will slip out of the needle hub causing malposition. The physician should be notified if catheter displacement is suspected.

6. Never attempt to push a catheter back into the patient once it has slipped out.

7. Sutures that are loose or have come out should be replaced by the physician.

8. A catheter that has slipped out (but with the tip remaining in good position) needs to be anchored with STERI-STRIPS or another suture to prevent further movement, particularly during dressing changes.

9. If a catheter is placed in an area of hair growth, the area should be shaved when necessary and scrubbed with a povidone-iodine solution.

10. The junction at the catheter hub and extension tubing on the single lumen catheter is considered sterile; therefore, this area is included under the dressing. Contaminants at this junction can seed down the catheter and enter the bloodstream. Luer lock connections will prevent the tubing from coming apart, so there is no need to keep the hub outside of the dressing.

D. PN Solutions

1. The PN solution should be inspected for small cracks, turbidity or precipitates and returned to the pharmacy if any are found.

2. The fat emulsion bottle should be checked for "oiling out," or separation of components, and returned to the pharmacy if this is found.

3. Do not infuse a PN solution through a peripheral vein if the final glucose concentration is higher than 10% in adults or 12.5% in infants.

4. Fat emulsions 10% and 20% may be infused centrally or peripherally, since they are isotonic.
5. Additions to the PN solution must be done prior to the initiation of the infusion in either the IV Room or in the inpatient pharmacies under well controlled sterile conditions.
6. The PN solution should never be used for dilution purposes when administering medications. When the line absolutely has to be used for medications or additional IV fluids, central PN should be stopped, and peripheral PN solution should be administered to decrease the risk of catheter sepsis. For data on physical and chemical incompatibilities, please refer to Section VIII C or page the PEN Team. If no data is available, it should be assumed the medication is incompatible.
7. Fat emulsion is the only fluid that should be infused with central PN.
8. If the PN solution is rendered unusable, dextrose 10% should be infused until the PN solution can be replaced.
9. Unused PN solutions expire in 24 hours and should be returned to the Central Pharmacy.
10. PN solution and fat emulsion bottles expire 24 hours after being hung and must be discontinued regardless of the amount remaining in the bottle.

E. Ordering PN: The 24-Hour PN Day

1. All PN orders must be written by 9:00 p.m. the evening before infusion for all hospitals.
2. All PN orders will be compounded and delivered to each nursing unit by:
   a. 1:00 p.m. for adults in University Hospital
   b. 9:00 a.m. for neonates, children, and adults in Mott, Women's and Holden Hospitals.
3. The PN solution is numbered sequentially from initiation of therapy until PN is discontinued.
4. The 24 hour PN day starts and finishes at:
   a. 2:00 p.m. for the University Hospital
   b. 10:00 a.m. for Mott, Women's and Holden Hospitals.
5. PN solutions will not be compounded after 4:00 p.m. in the University Hospital and after 6:00 a.m. in Mott, Women's and Holden Hospitals.

F. Tubing

1. The IV administration set, filter and extension tubing must be changed every 72 hours. This should be done at 2:00 p.m. (10:00 a.m. in Mott) when the PN solution is being changed. The lipid tubing must be changed every 24 hours.
2. Vented tubing is necessary for bottles, but not for plastic bags.
3. Stopcocks are not to be connected to the PN line except under life threatening circumstances.
4. All tubing junctions in Mott Hospital should be taped.
5. After careful cleaning of the Y-port below the filter with an alcohol swab, the primed fat emulsion line should be inserted with a 23 gauge, one-inch needle into the Y-port. Secure with a three-inch wide piece of tape.

G. Filters

1. Filters are used to remove particulate matter, air and pathogens from the line.
2. The filter should be changed at the same time the PN solution and tubing are changed, i.e., every 72 hours.
3. Fat emulsion must not be infused through a filter. It must be administered via the Y-port below the filter.
4. If the filter breaks, cracks or is clogged inadvertently with fat emulsion, immediately remove it to prevent possible clotting of the central line. Replace it as soon as possible.
5. If leaking, cracking or separation from the IV tubing occurs, check for the following problem areas:
   a. Kink or clot distal to the filter?
   b. Has the fat emulsion inadvertently clogged the filter?
   c. Has the filter been changed within the past 72 hours?

H. Infusion Pumps

1. Central and peripheral PN solutions should be administered by means of an infusion device according to the Nursing policy and Procedure Protocol #62-03-005.
2. Time-taping the PN solution is still necessary with an infusion pump. Not taping may foster reliance on machinery that can occasionally malfunction.

I. Flow Rates

1. Do not attempt to "catch up".
2. Notify the physician if there are mechanical or other difficulties that alter the rate of flow by an amount greater than 10%.
3. The flow rate will need to be increased if peripheral PN is being interrupted for IVPB medications. Contact the PEN Team for recommendations.
4. PN solutions routinely contain more than 1000 mL; therefore, there is no need to wait until the PN solution is completely empty before changing it.
5. At the initiation of PN therapy, the solution should be infused slowly to allow pancreatic adjustment to the increased glucose load. PN should be discontinued slowly for the same reasons. Note the glucose concentration of the solution prior to administration. The more concentrated solutions (greater than 35%) should be started at a rate no greater than 30 mL/hr.

J. Charting

1. Insertion of a central venous catheter, its location and any complications should be documented in the patient's record.
2. Drainage or redness at the insertion site, skin breakdown or catheter irregularities should be documented.
3. Administration of PN should be charted on the IV administration record or 24 hour flow sheet. PN solution number(s) and the time and date of administration should be recorded. This sheet becomes a permanent part of the patient's record. Unused PN solutions should also be charted.
4. Administration of a daily heparin flush solution (100 units/mL) to maintain the patency of unused, multilumen ports should be recorded on the medication record. Include the name of the drug, the amount and frequency of administration.

K. Nursing Policies

The following policies have been approved by the Nursing Practice Committee of the University of Michigan Hospitals.

1. Luer lock extension tubing **must** be attached to all central catheters.
2. Only physicians may remove central venous catheters.
3. When indicated, using aseptic technique, nurses may:
   a. Aspirate air or a clot from a central venous catheter.
   b. **Gently** irrigate a central catheter with normal saline using a TB syringe.
4. Nurses should not attempt to remove a kink from a central catheter if it causes any part of the catheter to be pushed back into the patient.

L. Measures to Minimize PN Solution Waste

Please call and inform Pharmacy IV Room in the University Hospital (6-8244) or Mott Pharmacy (4-8208) if:

1. PN has been discontinued on a patient.
2. The patient has been transferred to another unit.
3. The PN solution cannot be located or is unusable.

X. RECOMMENDED MONITORING FOR ADULTS

A. Variables to be Monitored

1. Blood Values

	Initial	2 x Weekly	Weekly	As Indicated
Hgb, Hct, WBC	X		X	
Total lymphocytes	X			X
Serum electrolytes	X			
Na, K, Cl, CO_2		X		
BUN, creatinine	X	X		
Ca, PO_4	X	X		
Total protein, albumin	X	X		
Glucose	X	X		
Liver enzymes: SGOT, SGPT, LDH, Alk Phos,	X	X		
Bilirubin D/T	X	X		
Mg	X		X	
Triglycerides	X		X	X
PT, PTT	X			X
Platelets	X			X
Fe, TIBC				X
Transferrin (may be estimated from TIBC)				X

2. Other Monitoring Measurements

a. General

	q Shift	Daily	As Indicated
Volume of infusate	X		
Oral intake	X		
Urine output, ostomy output, fistula, NG	X		
Weight		X	
Height			Initial
Temperature	X		
Anthropometric measurements			X
Skin Tests: PPD, Candida, Mumps			X

b Urine

	q Shift	Daily	As Indicated
Glucose		X	
Specific gravity		X	
24-hour UUN			X

c. Catheter Data

	q Shift	Daily	As Indicated
Route and date placed, chest film confirmation of position			Initial
			X
Date removed and reasons for removal			X
Catheter tip cultures			X
Blood cultures			X

B. Patient Responses

- If weight gain is one of the goals for the patient on PN, an increase of ½% of total body weight per day or up to ¼ to ½ pound per day (approximately 0.2 kg/d) should be expected. A greater weight gain than this suggests accumulation of excess fluid or increased fat stores.
- Stool frequency and amount is lessened while the patient is on total parenteral nutrition.
- Hallucinations of taste and smell may develop the longer the patient is NPO. The patient may become unduly preoccupied with food and/or become angry and sleepy at mealtime.
- PN may suppress appetite, and the patient should be reassured that appetite will eventually return when the PN is tapered and stopped.
- Protein synthesis depends in part on the patient's activity level. Physical exercise is essential for adequate regeneration of skeletal muscle, and physical therapy should not be neglected.
- Patients with severe diseases or metabolic complications will require more frequent monitoring of laboratory and clinical variables.
- Adult patients may develop elevated LFT's on PN (SGOT, SGPT, alkaline phosphatase, bilirubin). Typically, these changes occur after one to three weeks and are transient, and return to baseline one to three weeks after PN is stopped. All patients developing elevated LFT's should be evaluated for the appropriateness of the PN regimen components (dextrose, fat emulsion, amino acids) and total caloric requirements.

XI. COMPLICATIONS RELATED TO PARENTERAL NUTRITION

Numerous complications associated with PN therapy have been reported and are described under the following four subheadings: technical complications, metabolic complications, respiratory failure and septic complications. These complications are most often minimized or prevented when recommended administration, monitoring, and catheter care guidelines are followed.

A. Technical Complications

Only physicians well experienced in the techniques of subclavian and internal jugular venipunctures should insert catheters for purposes of parenteral nutrition. PN catheter insertion is never an emergency, and should only be done under planned circumstances with sufficient help available and with careful attention to aseptic technique. (Please refer to the section "Central Venous Catheter Insertion Guidelines"). Possible complications at the time of catheter insertion may include:

Pneumothorax	Thromboembolism
Hemothorax	Catheter embolism
Hydromediastinum	Catheter malposition
Subclavian artery	Thoracic duct laceration
puncture	Cardiac perforation and tamponade
Subclavian hematoma	Brachial plexus injury
Innominate or Subclavian	Horner's Syndrome
vein laceration	Phrenic nerve paralysis
Carotid artery injury	Air embolism

Even with experienced hands and under the best circumstances, a small but finite number of complications may occur. Pneumothorax is the most prevalent complication of subclavian venipuncture, occurring in up to 5% of attempted catheterizations. The pneumothorax may be asymptomatic and resolve or may require needle aspiration or (tube) thoracostomy. Instructing the patient to hold his breath on deep expiration or temporarily stopping positive pressure mechanical ventilation will reduce the incidence of pneumothorax. A chest film is **mandatory** after every catheterization or replacement of a catheter over a guidewire. A chest film will alert the physician to the possible occurrence of one of several of the above listed complications and will confirm the satisfactory position of the catheter before initiating PN infusion.

Puncture of the subclavian artery is the next most frequent complication and can be minimized by maintaining the angle of entry as close to the horizontal plane as possible. If arterial blood is returned on insertion of the catheter trocar needle, the needle should be withdrawn and direct pressure applied for a minimum of five minutes.

Puncture of the carotid artery is the most common complication of percutaneous internal jugular vein catheterization. When this complication occurs, pressure applied directly to the puncture site alone is sufficient. If this complication is unrecognized, however, the resulting hematoma of the neck may lead to tracheal compression and respiratory compromise.

Air embolism is a potentially fatal complication of percutaneous catheterization of the subclavian and internal jugular veins. To minimize the occurrence of this complication, the patient should be placed in a Trendelenberg position during the removal of the syringe from the needle trocar and passage of the catheter into the vein. Alternatively, the transition should be made rapidly during deep expiration or with mechanical ventilation temporarily interrupted. A second increased risk of introduction of air into the venous system is during routine tubing changes. The Nursing Practice Manual outlines those points which should minimize this complication. If a patient becomes inadvertently disconnected from his intravenous tubing, or the physician suspects the introduction of air during attempted subclavian or internal jugular vein catheter insertion, the immediate management should consist of clamping off the catheter or the tubing, and placing the patient with his left side down in the Trendelenberg position. If the catheter is in place, an attempt should be made to aspirate the air. Fresh sterile tubing should be connected to the catheter hub. If the tubing becomes disconnected above the filter, the filter itself will act as an air lock and prevent the patient from siphoning air into the vascular system.

B. Metabolic Complications

The metabolic complications outlined below include only the more common complications related to glucose, acid-base and electrolyte imbalances. These complications can be detected early or avoided altogether by regular and thoughtful monitoring of the patient according to the protocol in the "Recommended Monitoring," Chapter X.

1. Hyperglycemia

It is recommended that PN therapy be initiated gradually as described in "Administration and Discontinuation of Parenteral Nutrition Solutions" Chapter VIII, Section F, in order to prevent hyperglycemia.

An elevated blood sugar may appear during initial PN therapy and is best not treated if it does not result in 4+ glucosuria or in a significant osmotic diuresis. Endogenous insulin secretion normally adjusts as the PN rate or concentration is increased over a 48- to 72-hour period and the blood glucose level returns to normal. For this reason, insulin should not be added to PN solutions routinely. If insulin therapy is required as judged by 4+ glucosuria, a blood sugar greater than 200 mg %, or a significant osmotic diuresis, regular human insulin should be added directly to the PN solution by the pharmacy as ordered by the primary physician. Initial dosage is usually 10 units per liter in adults and may be increased as necessary. Alternatively, a sliding scale insulin coverage regimen or an intravenous insulin infusion may be used to gain control of elevated glucose. Then when glucose control is maintained, the appropriate amount of insulin can be added to the PN solution. Patients stable on PN who suddenly develop a blood sugar greater than 200 mg %, or who require increasing insulin, should be worked up for other causes of this finding, particularly sepsis. Unexplained and sudden glucose intolerance may frequently be the first sign of systemic sepsis which might not otherwise be apparent for several hours by the traditional signs, such as fever, chills, tachycardia or hypotension.

Hyperglycemia and persistent glucosuria producing osmotic diuresis is the etiology of the extreme complication of hyperosmolar, hyperglycemic nonketotic dehydration, which is frequently accompanied by deteriorating mental status and coma. Blood and urine assays do not show the presence of ketone bodies, and metabolic acidosis is generally present (in contradistinction to diabetic keto-acidosis). This condition can progress rapidly to death if not treated immediately by stopping the hypertonic infusion, hydrating with large amounts of hypotonic solution and administering intravenous insulin with careful monitoring. There may also be potassium and sodium abnormalities requiring correction.

The patient undergoing a major surgical operation frequently becomes less glucose tolerant because of endogenous hormone secretion. Therefore, we recommend that the PN infusion rate be routinely decreased by a factor of one half when the patient is taken to the operating room. The infusion can usually be brought back to the preoperative rate within 48 hours after surgery, provided the blood glucose concentration has remained within an acceptable range during and just after the operation.

Since the use of insulin in infants is quite complicated and the risk of blood sugar of 200 to 300 mg % is not great, we do not recommend instituting insulin therapy in this age group until the blood sugar exceeds 300 mg %.

2. Hypoglycemia

The most frequent cause of hypoglycemia in patients receiving parenteral nutrition is a sudden cessation or reduction in the rate of PN infusion. Symptoms, such as diaphoresis, confusion, or agitation, in a patient receiving PN should alert the physician that hypoglycemia may be present. Symptomatic hypoglycemia should be managed initially with a bolus administration of 50% dextrose. Further management is dictated by serum glucose and clinical response. When the PN solution must be discontinued or has run out, administration of 10% dextrose in water will prevent symptomatic hypoglycemia.

3. Hyperkalemia

Patients receiving PN may develop an abnormally elevated serum potassium if they are not adequately anabolic and, therefore, are unable to fully utilize the administered potassium. Other causes of hyperkalemia include decreased renal function, low cardiac output, tissue necrosis, and systemic sepsis. Potassium should be reduced or withheld from the PN solution until the underlying problem is resolved. Severe symptomatic hyperkalemia should be treated in the usual way with bicarbonate, glucose and insulin intravenously, and intravenous calcium for any serious cardiotoxic effects.

4. Hypokalemia

As a patient on PN becomes anabolic and begins to synthesize new protein, there is an obligatory requirement for intracellular potassium. Therefore, doses of intravenous potassium in PN solution of at least 40 mEq/L are required for the adult. It is not unusual for this requirement to reach 200 mEq of potassium per day, and this will become evident if the patient's serum potassium is monitored on a regular basis.

5. Hypercalcemia-Hypermagnesemia-Hyperphosphatemia

Depressed central nervous system activity and muscle weakness out of proportion to the patient's illness may indicate elevated calcium, magnesium or phosphorus levels. Because of an increased catabolic state, the amount of calcium, magnesium and phosphorus included in the PN solution may not be fully utilized. If increased catabolism or decreased renal function occur, the concentration of these ions should be decreased and the need for them assessed on a day-to-day basis.

6. Hypocalcemia

   Malnourished and debilitated patients frequently have a decrease in total serum albumin and a proportionately low calcium (approximately a 0.8 mg decrease in calcium per g drop in albumin). Since the free, ionized calcium is normal, it is unlikely that this hypocalcemia would be symptomatic with paresthesias, confusion, positive Chvostek sign and tetany. However, the standard amount of calcium (4.5 mEq) should be included in the PN solution. If additional amounts are necessary, these can be ordered within the limitations of solubility.

7. Hypomagnesemia

   Magnesium is required during increasing anabolism and protein synthesis in the same fashion as potassium and phosphorus. Hallucination, vertigo, ileus, and hyperreflexia may indicate hypomagnesemia, and additional amounts of magnesium sulfate can be added to the PN solution.

8. Hypophosphatemia

   Phosphate is required intracellularly for high energy phosphate compounds; phospholipids participate in membrane structure, and phosphorus is necessary for bone synthesis and a number of other physiologic and biochemical processes. It is not surprising, therefore, that hypophosphatemia may result during increased anabolism. Symptoms include mental deterioration and lethargy, which may progress to convulsive seizures and coma. Hemolysis, thrombocytopenia, and other dysfunctions of erythrocytes, platelets, and leukocytes have been reported. Metabolic acidosis, respiratory failure and a congestive cardiomyopathy may develop. The consequences of profound phosphorus depletion has been reported to lead to acute cardiopulmonary decompensation and death. The daily requirement for phosphate may increase substantially during PN, and an additional amount of phosphate should be added to the daily PN regimen according to the protocol in Chapter VIII. This is especially important in the neonate and infant whose phosphate requirements are much higher than in an adult. Phosphate is available as a potassium or sodium salt. Therefore, it is important to specify which salt is desired when ordering additional phosphate in PN solutions.

9. Hypertriglyceridemia

   Although lipid levels in the serum remain normal or slightly elevated during PN which includes fat emulsion, occasionally serum triglycerides may rise significantly. In this situation, the rate of fat administration should be appropriately reduced, or fat should be administered on an every two to three day schedule. Perhaps the most frequently observed effects after long term administration of fat are the moderate elevation of liver enzymes and the deposition of intravenous fat pigment in Kupffer's cells. These deposits do not appear to affect liver function. Intravenous fat emulsions are contraindicated in patients with pathologic hyperlipemia, lipid nephrosis, or acute pancreatitis if accompanied by hyperlipemia.

10. Hypercapnia (Respiratory Failure)

Infusion of PN solutions with high dextrose content or infusion of calories in excess of patient's needs can compromise respiratory function in patients with chronic obstructive pulmonary disease by causing increased CO_2 production. This problem is often apparent in unsuccessful attempts to wean patients from ventilatory support. The increased CO_2 production causes increased ventilatory requirements by stimulating an increase in minute ventilation. In patients with compromised respiratory function, there is limited alveolar reserve and therefore, less efficient CO_2 excretion. If the patient is being overfed, total calories should be reduced to meet estimated needs. The PN solution can be modified to provide sufficient calories, yet minimize CO_2 production, by decreasing the dextrose concentration and providing increased calories as fat (up to 60% of total calories provided). Indirect calorimetry measurements are very helpful in these patients and are performed by the Critical Care Diagnostic Service (936-5860)

11. Refeeding Syndrome

Refeeding severely malnourished patients requires caution when using hypertonic dextrose solutions. Initiation of aggressive nutritional support will result in intracellular trapping of phosphate, resulting in a drop of serum phosphate and possible respiratory failure in patients previously utilizing body fat stores as their predominant fuel source. Additionally, when refed too rapidly, potassium and magnesium shift intracellularly, causing pronounced hypokalemia and hypomagnesemia. Nutrient delivery should begin with the patient's basal energy requirements (approximately 28 kcal/kg/day) and should be advanced gradually over a 5-7 day period. Serum K, PO_4, and Mg should be monitored daily during the first week of therapy. Excessive fluid loads should be minimized to avoid an increased cardiac workload leading to congestive heart failure.

12. Trace Element Deficiency

Zinc deficiency during long-term PN has been well documented in children and adults. It is usually manifested by hair loss, seborrheic dermatitis around the nose and mouth, and occasionally ileus. Chromium deficiency, although very rare, can produce a diabetes-like syndrome; and copper deficiency results in hypochromic, normocytic anemia and neutropenia. Selenium deficiency, a potential complication of long term PN support, is manifested by muscular pain and cardiomyopathy. Although rare, molybdenum deficiency manifested by neurologic abnormalities, absence of urinary inorganic sulfate, hypermethionemia, hypouricemia and hyperuricosuria, may also occur among long term PN supported patients. In order to avoid these complications, a trace element solution should be administered with the PN solution on a daily basis. Levels of trace elements, not routinely provided to the long term PN patients, should be assessed periodically.

C. Septic Complications

1. General Considerations

Septic complications in a patient receiving PN are suggested by varying combinations of temperature elevation, sudden glucose intolerance, hypotension, oliguria or a general deterioration in clinical condition.

Considerations of PN initiation in a febrile patient are as follows:
a. PN is **never** an emergency procedure. A febrile patient should have a reasonable investigation of the source of fever prior to initiating PN.
b. PN should not be initiated during the early stages of an **uncontrolled** infection and particularly during recurrent septicemia.
c. If PN is initiated while a patient is febrile, periodic blood cultures should be done while the patient remains febrile (i.e., every 2 - 4 days).

2. Protocol for Workup of Possible Catheter Sepsis:
a. Investigate all possible sources of infection (i.e., lung, GU, abdomen, wounds, sputum, urine). If the catheter site reveals evidence of infection (e.g., purulence) remove the catheter.
b. If no other septic source for the above complications is found after 24 hours of investigation, remove catheter.
c. Draw quantitative blood cultures (for aerobes, anaerobes and "hold for fungi") through the catheter and from one peripheral site. Once the blood culture is obtained, the catheter should be removed or changed over a guidewire; the catheter should also be cultured (see 2.f.).
d. Multilumen catheters should be removed as soon as possible in favor of a single lumen catheter. Unless the exit site is infected, removal may be done over a guidewire using aseptic technique.
e. If the PN solution is suspected, the entire infusion setup (with a sterile needle capping the distal tubing) should be sent to the Microbiology Laboratory for culture for aerobes, anaerobes, and fungi. It should be replaced with new IV tubing and PN solutions or 10% dextrose water.
f. To culture the catheter: prep skin; remove catheter and with sterile scissors cut off 2 one-inch pieces into a sterile test tube and 1 one-inch piece into a Cary-Blair anaerobic transport tube and send to Microbiology for aerobic, anaerobic, and fungal cultures.
g. If the catheter is removed because of a strong suspicion of catheter sepsis, wait 24 hours before reinsertion (if possible). If the catheter must be replaced earlier, wait 6 hours after appropriate broad spectrum antibiotics are begun, and reinsert at a different site.

3. Absolute Indications for Catheter Removal
a. Septic shock (prior to culture results).
b. Laboratory proven bacteremia or fungemia.
c. Focal infection at site of catheter insertion.
d. Embolic phenomena.
e. Persistent fever with no other source found.

XII. PEDIATRIC PARENTERAL NUTRITION

A. General Recommendations

Several special considerations make parenteral nutrition in the premature neonate, the infant, and young child significantly different from that in the adult. These relate to smaller body size, rapid growth, highly variable fluid requirements, and in newborn infants, the immaturity of certain organ systems. An infant or child stressed by major infection, severe trauma, or major surgery, is frequently unable to tolerate enteral nutrition. Inadequate nutritional support may result in weakening of respiratory muscles, depression of central nervous system function, apnea, increased difficulty in weaning from mechanical ventilation, and increased susceptibility to infection.

Because of the potentially severe problems that may result from malnutrition, parenteral nutrition should be initiated as early as possible when a physician determines that an infant or small child is malnourished or unlikely to tolerate enteral nutrition within a three to five day period. Most normal newborns establish positive nitrogen balance with weight stabilization or weight gain by the second to fourth postpartum day. In infants unable to take adequate enteral nutrition, sufficient nutrients can usually be provided with peripheral parenteral nutrition by infusing glucose-amino acid solutions concomitantly with fat emulsion. Central venous access may be required in infants who require fluid restriction, or in infants with limited peripheral vein access and with the need for prolonged parenteral nutrition.

Every infant receiving parenteral nutrition goes through a period of physiologic adjustment which can be divided into two stages. The first stage is a time of increasing tolerance to the PN solution as reflected by the serum and urine glucose levels. During this time the glucose and lipid dose should be gradually increased until a sufficient number of calories are provided or until other factors such as the volume of fluid tolerated, limit further increases. The time required for this initial adjustment phase is extremely variable. Immature infants, or those with severe stress due to infection or respiratory insufficiency, will require a longer period for stabilization than the more mature infant. The second stage marks the beginning of the period during which the infant is receiving an adequate number of calories for weight gain and electrolyte balance is stable. Optimal weight gain for newborns during this phase should be 15 to 25 grams per day, or 1/2% of total body weight in kg/day in older patients. Weight gain greater than this may reflect excess fluid administration and fluid retention. Inadequate weight gain may reflect an underlying metabolic insult, such as sepsis. During both phases, it is very important to keep accurate intake and output records, and obtain daily weights at the same time and with the same scale each day. Urine output should run 1 mL/kg/hour or more, with urine specific gravity between 1.005 and 1.015 in the absence of glucosuria.

B. Ordering Parenteral Nutrition Solutions

1. Neonates and infants up to 10 kg of body weight
   a. Order on the form:
      DAILY PARENTERAL NUTRITION (PN) ORDER AND ADMINISTRATION FORM FOR NEONATAL PATIENTS #H2060395 (Appendix E)

1) Follow the format on the front of the PN Form.
2) Sequence number of the PN formulation should be indicated for the duration the patient is supported with parenteral nutrition.
3) Total volume of PN solution should be ordered to last 24 hours. The pharmacy will automatically increase the volume ordered to account for the volume of the IV tubing.
4) Flow rate per hour should be specified.
5) Patient's weight must be provided for the prescription to be compounded.
6) Volume, amino acid, and all electrolytes should be ordered per kilogram.
7) Calcium-phosphate compatibility factor should be calculated for every order and adjusted to prevent precipitation.
8) Dextrose, amino acid, and fat emulsion calories along with the nonprotein-calories-to-gram-nitrogen ratio should be calculated to ensure the appropriate balance of PN components.
9) Additional specific prescribing information is on the back of the form and in Appendix E.
10) PN orders must be received by Pharmacy by 9:00 p.m. the night before the TPN is to be administered.

2. Pediatric patients up to 10 to 30 kg of body weight
   a. Non-standard and standard PN solutions for neonates and infants and adolescents from 10 to 30 kg of body weight can be ordered on the form: DAILY PARENTERAL NUTRITION (PN) ORDER AND ADMINISTRATION FORM FOR PEDIATRIC PATIENTS #H2060425 (Appendix D)
      1) Only one column on the order form for the appropriate formulation should be filled out, i.e., non-standard, peripheral or central formulation.
      2) Sequence number of the PN formulation should be indicated for the duration the patient is supported with parenteral nutrition.
      3) Total volume of PN solution should be ordered to last 24 hours.
      4) Flow rate per hour should be specified with consistent flow rates over a 24 hour period.
      5) Patient's weight must be provided for the prescription to be compounded.
      6) Fat emulsion should be ordered on the PN order form designating the desired percent emulsion and the flow rate.
      7) All electrolytes ordered should be per total volume.
   b. Non-Standard PN Formulations
      1) Order non-standard formulations for pediatric patients only when none of the standard formulations meet the patient's requirements.
      2) Addition of one or more ingredients to a standard formulation is permissible, provided that the quantities of such electrolytes meet the compatibility guidelines (Chapter VIII, Section C).
      3) If the non-standard solution is ordered, amino acids should be ordered in grams, and dextrose should be ordered in percent final volume.
      4) See Table 7 and Appendix E for prescribing information.

c. Standard Central Formulation

This formulation should be prescribed for patients with a central venous line only. The profile of this solution is as follows:

Standard Central Parenteral Nutrition Formulation

Amino Acids (3.5%)	35	g	**Approximate Volume**
Dextrose (25%)	250	g	1050 mL
Calcium	9	mEq	**Approximate Osmolarity**
Magnesium	5	mEq	1750 mOsm/L
Potassium	40	mEq	**Total Caloric Value**
Sodium	35	mEq	990 kcal
Acetate	82	mEq	(approx. 1 kcal/mL)
Chloride	35	mEq	**Nitrogen Content**
Phosphorus	12	mM	5.5 g
Heparin	1000	units	**Non-Protein Calorie/g Nitrogen**
Pediatric Multivitamins	3	mL	155:1

Pediatric trace elements will be automatically added to all PN solutions ordered at a dose of 0.1 mL/kg/day unless otherwise indicated by the physician.

d. Standard Peripheral Formulation

The profile of this formulation is as follows:

Standard Peripheral Parenteral Nutrition Formulation*

Amino Acids (2.0%)	20	g	**Approximate Volume**
Dextrose (10%)	100	g	1050 mL
Calcium	9	mEq	**Approximate Osmolarity**
Magnesium	5	mEq	810 mOsm/L
Potassium	30	mEq	**Total Caloric Value**
Sodium	35	mEq	420 kcal
Acetate	60	mEq	(approx. 0.4 kcal/mL)
Chloride	35	mEq	**Nitrogen Content**
Phosphorus	6	mM	3.1 g
Heparin Sodium	1000	units	**Non-Protein Calorie/g Nitrogen**
Pediatric Multivitamins	3	mL	85:1

Pediatric trace elements will be automatically added to all PN solutions ordered at a dose of 0.1 mL/kg/day unless otherwise indicated by the physician.

*Due to the high osmolarity of this peripheral solution it should be infused concurrently with fat emulsion.

3. Adolescents over 30 kg of body weight

This patient population is handled in a fashion similar to the adult population.

a. Standard PN Formulation should be ordered on the form:

DAILY PARENTERAL NUTRITION (PN) ORDER AND ADMINISTRATION FORM FOR STANDARD FORMULATION FOR ADOLESCENT AND ADULT PATIENTS #H-2060413 (Appendix B)

b. Non-Standard PN Formulations should be ordered on the form:

DAILY PARENTERAL NUTRITION (PN) ORDER AND ADMINISTRATION FORM FOR ADOLESCENT AND ADULT PATIENTS #H-2060401 (Appendix C)

For detailed prescribing information see Chapter VIII on Parenteral Nutrition for Adolescent and Adult Patients.

C. Administering Parenteral Nutrition Solutions

In general, infants should be started on half-strength solutions (4-8 mg/kg/min of dextrose) and advanced to 3/4 and full-strength (10-14 mg/kg/min maximum) over the ensuing 24 to 48 hours, depending on urine and blood glucose determinations. Total volume can then be increased as tolerated to further increase caloric intake (see Tables 8 & 9). Because of the high rate of phlebitis with hypersmolar solutions, peripheral PN concentration should not exceed 12.5% dextrose and 2.5% amino acids.

In low birth weight and critically ill infants, umbilical artery (UAC) and vein (UVC) catheters are usually present. Central strength formulations (greater than 10%) can be infused through a UVC once placement of the catheter tip above the diaphragm is confirmed. Concentrations of dextrose administered through a UAC should usually be limited to a maximum of 12.5%.

Studies show it is safe to begin fat emulsion at a rate of .5-1 g/kg/day on the first day of TPN. Lipids can be advanced at a rate of .5 g/kg/day to a maximum of 3 g/kg/day in premature infants, and 4 g/kg/day in full term infants.

Central PN solutions may be administered alone, or concomitantly with intravenous fat. Peripheral formulations are generally given concomitantly with intravenous fat to reduce the osmolarity of the final solution and keep the total volume within manageable limits. Ideally, the daily intravenous calorie budget should approximate normal calorie distribution in a balanced diet: 50% carbohydrate, 40% fat and 10% protein. In actual practice, only enough fat need be given to prevent essential fatty acid deficiency. Most importantly, the sum of the nonprotein calories should be sufficient to provide a total nonprotein-calorie-to-grams-of-nitrogen ratio in the range of 150:1 to 300:1. This range is necessary to achieve the optimal utilization and protein-sparing effect of the administered PN solution. Excessive or unbalanced protein intake has been associated with metabolic acidosis in small premature infants.

Table 7 is designed to provide a guide for parenteral nutrition in newborn infants and small children. The nutritional requirements for children over age 3 years and teenagers will not be dealt with separately except to reiterate their increased caloric requirements due to rapid growth and development. In addition, each pediatric unit or service may have guidelines for specific application of PN for problems unique to their patients. Further assistance is available through the PEN Team office.

D. Monitoring

Infants on PN must be carefully monitored. In addition to accurate daily intake, output, weight, and weekly length and head circumference, judicious use of blood tests is very important in infants and children due to their small total blood volume. Table 10 outlines recommended tests and frequency of monitoring. Careful attention to the values will alert the physician to potential metabolic complications (outlined in subsequent pages and in Chapter XI) and ensure optimal benefit from PN therapy.

E. Complications

1. Technical complications

The incidence of technical complications due to placement and position of central lines in infants and children has been greatly reduced in recent years by careful attention to aseptic technique and x-ray check after catheter insertion. The introduction of non-reactive silicone catheters in place of polyvinylchloride catheters has reduced the incidence of foreign body reaction and subclavian vein or vena cava thrombosis. The incidence of cardiac arrhythmias due to irritation from the catheter has been greatly reduced by placing the tip of the catheter at the junction of the superior vena cava and the right atrium rather than in the heart. Suturing the catheter to the skin at the catheter-cutaneous junction and checking to be sure that the catheter is secure at each 72 hour dressing change has greatly reduced the frequency of catheter dislocation. The complications arising from administration of PN through an umbilical artery catheter (UAC) in neonates are associated with the UAC placement, e.g., vasospasm, thrombosis, embolization, hypertension, hemorrhage, and necrotizing enterocolitis. A list and short discussion of common technical complications at the time of catheter insertion is presented in Chapter XI, Section A.

Almost all of the technical complications inherent in central PN can be avoided by use of peripheral PN administration. Phlebitis and superficial skin slough are the most common complications in patients receiving peripheral PN. The incidence of phlebitis is reduced in patients receiving concomitant intravenous fat emulsion. Simultaneous infusion of fat reduces the osmolarity and increases the pH of the PN solution, and although still slightly hypertonic, the fat emulsion appears to protect the vein from phlebitis. If an infiltrated IV site is identified quickly, it is usually benign, and the extravasated fluid is rapidly reabsorbed. This process is enhanced by warm, moist dressings to the area and silver sulfadiazine dressings in those few cases where skin slough occurs. Very rarely a skin slough site will require skin grafting.

2. Metabolic Complications

Almost every conceivable metabolic complication has been reported during total parenteral nutrition. Table 11 lists the more common metabolic complications, and although serious consequences may ensue if metabolic complications go undetected for any length of time, careful clinical monitoring and appropriate adjustment of the PN solution results in most patients tolerating parenteral nutrition infusion quite well.

Hyperglycemia is most common in the low birth weight or premature infant, during the first 24 hours postoperatively, or in the presence of systemic sepsis. Once sepsis has been ruled out, or effectively treated, hyperglycemia usually responds to diluting the PN solution and gradually increasing the concentration again to full strength over 24 to 48 hours. If hyperglycemia cannot be controlled by this simple manipulation, then insulin may be added to the PN solution. Nondiabetic infants and children rarely require added insulin.

Hypoglycemia has been reported when PN is abruptly terminated. $D_{10}W$ should always be hung when central PN solution is interrupted for any reason. The PN infusion should be gradually tapered when nutrition by vein is no longer required. Hypoglycemia normally does not occur when peripheral PN is interrupted, and no special actions or monitoring need be taken.

Metabolic acidosis is historically associated with the metabolism of protein hydrolysates containing large proportions of chloride salts. The advent of crystalline amino acid solutions which contain similar proportions of acetate and chloride salts have decreased the incidence of metabolic acidosis related to the TPN solution. Administration of chloride in amounts greater than 6 mEq/kg/day, and administration of excessive protein loads are also associated with metabolic acidosis. Premature infants and patients with kidney or liver disease are at increased risk of developing acidosis with PN, and frequent monitoring of serum electrolytes and blood pH are indicated.

Hyperlipidemia secondary to the use of large amounts of fat emulsions in the neonate could potentially lead to displacement of albumin-bound bilirubin by free fatty acids and thereby augment hyperbilirubinemia. In general the use of fat emulsions should be curtailed only when the serum bilirubin is near exchange transfusion levels. Hyperlipidemia is also associated with impaired immune function, fat overload syndrome, and other potentially long-term complications, such as arterial sclerosis. Serum triglycerides should be monitored, especially after increasing the dose, and lipids held if the level is greater than 250 mg %.

Essential fatty acid deficiency may manifest itself as a desquamating generalized red skin rash that occurs after a 7-10 day period of fat-free PN. A minimum of four percent of daily caloric requirements provided as linoleic acid in an intravenous fat emulsion will prevent essential fatty acid deficiency.

Hypo/hypercalcemia, as well as **hypo/hyperphosphatemia** have all been reported in patients receiving parenteral nutrition. This occurs when inappropriate amounts of calcium and phosphorus are added to the PN solution and can be avoided by careful calculation and monitoring of the serum calcium and phosphorus. Premature infants require relatively more calcium than full term infants, and most pediatric patients should receive at least 1 mM phosphorus/kg/day in the PN infusate.

Hypomagnesemia is usually associated with patients suffering from severe diarrhea. Low magnesium can lead to ileus, hyperreflexia, and eventually seizures. Like potassium and phosphorus, larger quantities of magnesium are required during increased anabolism and protein synthesis that result from PN therapy.

Copper and zinc deficiencies have also been observed in patients with chronic diarrhea or in patients with inadequate amounts of trace elements present in their PN regimen. Patients receiving the recommended trace element solution are unlikely to develop deficiency syndromes unless abnormal losses persist.

Cholestatic jaundice attributed to PN is more common in premature infants than in older children or adults. Cholestasis may be related to the immaturity of the biliary excretory system in the infant, coupled with an incomplete understanding of the proper amino acid mixture for premature infants. This occurs typically after 2-3 weeks of TPN administration. In some premature infants, TPN-associated cholestasis has persisted for weeks to months and has been associated with fibrosis and death. Although abnormalities in liver function, such as elevations in SGOT, LDH, and direct bilirubin, have frequently been reported within 2-14 days after beginning parenteral nutrition, histological examination of the liver does not reveal any consistent pathological change, and the abnormalities generally return to normal once the PN therapy has been stopped. The abnormalities seen in patients receiving intravenous fat are essentially the same as those seen in fat-free PN regimens. Abnormal liver function tests accompanied by fever and increasing jaundice are indications to stop PN. Caloric overload may be partially responsible for liver toxicity in immature patients. The use of bedside indirect calorimetry to measure resting energy expenditure (REE) is helpful for estimating daily caloric needs, and may be important in avoiding overfeeding.

Peripheral eosinophilia, in the range of 5 to 10 percent, may develop in patients receiving fat emulsion. This appears to be of no clinical significance and resolves when the intravenous fat is stopped.

Metabolic bone disease has been observed in infants and children receiving long term parenteral nutrition. This condition is most often associated with deficiencies of calcium and phosphorus. Excessive amounts of Vitamin D, micronutrient deficiencies and accumulation of toxic substances in TPN solution also contribute. Signs of metabolic bone disease include bone pain, pathologic fractures, increased serum alkaline phosphatase, and a "washed-out" demineralized appearance on bone x-ray. Treatment of this malady includes maximizing calcium and phosphorus intake. Other therapies to be considered include deleting Vitamin D from the TPN solution. Please consult the PEN Team if this manipulation is required.

3. Infectious Complications

Sepsis continues to be the major complication of centrally infused parenteral nutrition in infants and children, and the protocol for work-up of possible catheter sepsis is the same as that described for the adult in Chapter XI. Placement of catheters under strict aseptic conditions and meticulous care of the catheter site with 72-hour standardized dressing changes will greatly reduce the incidence of septic complications. In addition, strict avoidance of the use of the PN catheter for blood drawing, administration of medication, or blood products, will minimize the risk of contamination and mechanical failure.

Peripheral PN administration has the advantage of eliminating most of the septic and technical complications inherent with central catheters. However, the avoidance of frequent infiltration and local infection or skin slough that may accompany peripheral IV infusion is dependent on the same careful attention to sterile technique of insertion and occlusive dressings that are important in central line management.

F. Pediatric Nutritional Assessment

Nutritional assessment of the pediatric patient differs from that of the adult. The pediatric patient, especially the infant, does not have the reserves of an adult and must be provided additional calories for growth. Thus, nutritional inadequacies are seen more quickly and can be more devastating in the pediatric age group. In addition to the biochemical parameters, such as albumin and total protein, body weight should be obtained daily, and height/length and head circumference should be measured at least weekly on all patients where adequate nutrient intake is questioned. (Refer to standardized growth charts for pediatric patients, Appendix K.) See Section IV for more complete nutritional assessment guidelines.

To estimate the caloric needs of the pediatric patient, please refer to Table 7. Resting Energy Expenditure (REE) for infants as well as for older children can be measured by indirect calorimetry which is obtainable by consulting the Metabolic Lab (936-5860) or Dr. John Wesley (764-6846). Clinical studies performed by our laboratory have determined that the best starting point for total daily calories in infants is REE + 45%. This allows for a weight gain of 15 - 25 g/day.

G. Pediatric Enteral Nutrition

Specialized enteral nutrition is indicated for the pediatric patient unable to ingest sufficient nutrients normally by mouth. The patient must have enough functional gut to absorb the formula administered. Successful introduction of enteric support requires appropriate formula selection and feeding regimen design.

1. Formula Selection

Three major categories of pediatric enteral products have been developed, based on the relative maturity of the child's GI tract, liver, and kidney function and age-specific nutrient requirements.

These categories include: a) formulas appropriate for premature infants, including breast milk, b) formulas appropriate for full term infants less than one year of age, and c) formulas appropriate for children one to six years of age, d) adult formulas are usually appropriate for children over six years of age.

a. Breast milk offers many actual and theoretical advantages and should be used whenever available. Because of variable amounts of protein available in breast milk and insufficient amounts of calcium and phosphorus, the use of supplements to breast milk should be considered in the VLBW infant. Premature infant formulas are also available and are specifically designed for infants that weigh less than 2 kg. The sources of carbohydrate, protein, and fat are tailored to meet the unique requirements of this population. Due to the decreased lactase levels seen in these patients, the lactose content has been reduced. The digestibility of the protein source has been improved by changing the whey: casein ratio to 60:40. Cysteine has been added and tyrosine has been reduced to provide a more appropriate amino acid composition. Premature infants have difficulty absorbing long chain fatty acids due to their reduced pool of bile acids. To improve fat absorption, all of these formulations contain a higher percentage of fat as medium chain triglycerides. Because of the increased demand for minerals for bone growth in the premature infant, selection of a formula high in calcium and phosphorus is recommended.

b. Full term infant formulas are appropriate for infants less than one year of age. Included in this category are cow's milk-based formulas, soy protein-based formulas, hypoallergenic protein hydrolysates and formulas with a modified fat source.

1) Cow's milk-based formulas have a nutrient distribution which closely approximates human milk. They are the formulas of choice in infants that do not have underlying GI disorders and are not breast fed. These formulas are available in concentrations of 20 and 24 kcal/ounce (0.66 and 0.8 kcal/mL).

2) Soy-based formulas are indicated when an allergy to the protein in cow's milk and/or lactose intolerance is diagnosed. All of these contain soy protein isolates as their protein source and are lactose free. The soy formulas are available in a concentration of 20 kcals/ounce (0.66 kcal/mL).

3) Hypoallergenic protein hydrolysate formulas are indicated in infants with cow's milk or other food allergies, severe/persistant diarrhea and other GI disturbances. They contain casein hydrolysates as their protein source, and a greater percentage of their fat is in the form of medium chain triglycerides.

4) Modified fat source formulas should be selected when significant steatorrhea occurs as in cystic fibrosis, intestinal resections, pancreatic insufficiency, biliary atresia and celiac disease. The majority of fat (83%) is in the form of medium chain triglycerides which requires no emulsification for absorption.

In addition to these full term infant formulas, specialized products for children with inborn errors of metabolism are available. For more information on these products, contact the Mott Clinical Nutritionists at 763-1531.

c. Formulas specifically designed for children between the ages of one to six years are currently commercially available. The pediatric formula, Pediasure, provides nutrients to meet or exceed the Recommended Dietary Allowances for this age group.

Appendix H details the easily crushable and liquid pediatric vitamin/mineral supplements and the modular products available at UMMC.

Categorization of the UMMC infant formulas is provided in Table 12. Nutrient composition of these formulas is detailed in Appendix G.

d. Guidelines outlined in Chapter XIII, Section F should be followed for enteral formula selection for children over six years of age.

2. Feeding Regimen Design

The preferred method of enteral feeding for children under one year of age is an intermittent regimen. This method most resembles nipple feeds and allows for the postprandial hormonal changes to occur. Generally the gastrointestinal tract will tolerate increases in volume before it will tolerate an increase in osmolarity. Small advances are made in volume followed by increases in concentration of the formula. The guidelines outlined below have been developed for the introduction of intermittent feedings.

a. Determine the child's energy, protein, vitamin, mineral, and fluid requirements for growth and maintenance.
b. Determine the volume of formula needed to meet these nutritional requirements. Divide this volume by the number of feedings to be given each day.
c. Initiate feedings at 1/4 to 1/2-strength formula of 10-15 mL/feeding (for premature infants start with 1-3 mL/feeding). Increase this volume by 2-10 mL increments each feeding as tolerated.
d. When the full desired volume per feeding is tolerated, the formula concentration is advanced to 3/4-strength for 24 hours and finally to full strength.

If intermittent feedings are not indicated, as when feeding directly into the small bowel, or if the patient is unable to tolerate bolus feedings, continuous drip feedings should be provided. Follow the guidelines outlined in Chapter XIII, Section F, to design a continuous feeding regimen.

TABLE 7 - PEDIATRIC PN

Component	Supplied As	Amount Required	Comments
Fluid	Combination of items below	60-150 mL/kg/day	See Tables 8 and 9. Monitor intake and output. Aim for urine output of 1-2 mL/kg/hr with urine Sp Gr. 1.005-1.015.
Calories	Protein 4.0 kcal/g CHO 3.4 kcal/g Fat 9.0 kcal/g (IV Fat emulsion 10% and 20%)	45-120 kcal/kg/day	Maintenance and Normal Growth Calorie requirement increased by any one of the following: 12% increase for each degree of fever above 37° C. 20-30% increase with major surgery 40-50% increase with severe sepsis 50-100% increase with long-term growth failure. *Premature infants should start at 80 kcal/kg and increase as needed for appropriate weight gain.
Protein	Amino Acid solution 5% 7%	To provide essential and nonessential amino acids 1.7-2.5 protein g/kg/day	In neonates, protein should be initiated at 1 g/kg and advanced to a maximum of 2.5 g/kg/day protein. For every gram of nitrogen provided, 150-300 nonprotein calories should be provided as carbohydrate or fat to maintain positive nitrogen balance. 1 g protein = 0.16 g nitrogen. See Appendix E for appropriate progression of protein based on non-protein calories for neonates.
Carbohydrate	D_5, D_{10}, D_{25}, D_{50}	To provide necessary calories Rate: 0.4-1.5 g/kg/hr.	Use D_{10} + $A_{2.0}$ for peripheral PN (0.4 kcal/mL) Nonprotein-calorie/gN ratio 85:1. Add fat emulsion for additional nonprotein calories. D_{25} + $A_{3.5}$ for Central PN (1.0 kcal/mL) Nonprotein-calorie/gN ratio 155:1. In neonates up to $D_{12.5}$ can be administered in peripheral lines and through umbilical artery catheters. D_{25} can be infused through umbilical venous catheters if proper line placement in the right atrium is confirmed.

Maintenance and Normal Growth table (Calories):

Age (yrs)	Kcal/kg
0-1*	90-120
1-7	75-90
7-12	60-75
12-18	45-60

TABLE 7 - PEDIATRIC PN Continued

Component	Supplied As	Amount Required	Comments
Fat	Fat emulsion 10% & 20%	To provide necessary calories 1-4 g/kg/day Rate: <.25 g/kg/hr.	Do not exceed 4 g/kg/day, (3.0 kg/day in premature infants), or approximately 50% of total calories; 4% of daily calories, given as linoleic acid from a fat emulsion, supplies the requirement for essential fatty acids. In neonates, 0.5 - 1 g/k/d of fat emulsion will meet this requirement.
			10% = 1.1 kcal/mL 20% = 2.0 kcal/mL
Na	NaCl; Na acetate Na phosphate	2-4 mEq/kg/day*	The acetate salt should be used in hyperchloremic patients. When used as a phosphate source, each millimole of Na phosphate provides approximately 1.3 mEq Na. Premature infants may have increased sodium needs.
K	KCl; K phosphate K acetate	2-4 mEq/kg/day*	Each millimole of K phosphate provides approximately 1.5 mEq potassium.
Ca	Ca Gluconate 10%	0.5-3.0 mEq/kg/day* 10 mL (1 g) provides 4.8 mEq	Premature infants require more calcium than full-term infants or children. An initial dose of 1 mEq/kg/day should be adjusted on basis of serum calcium and PO_4 measurements. Precipitation factor should be calculated when using a neonatal form and should not exceed a factor of 3. See Appendix E.
PO_4	K phosphate Na Phosphate	0.5-1.5 mM/kg/day*	Order only to provide maintenance phosphorus, the major anion of intracellular fluids, important in the formation of ATP, ADP, and creatine phosphate. Due to valence change with pH, PO_4 is ordered in millimoles rather than milliequivalents. The normal serum level for term newborns is 3.5 to 8.6 mg/dL; for premature newborns during the first week only it is 5.4-10.9 mg/dL, and declines toward term newborns in 3-4 weeks.
Mg	$MgSO_4$	0.5-1.0 mEq/kg/day*	A major cation in the body acting as a catalyst for many intracellular enzymatic reactions.

*Electrolyte ranges are for patients up to 10 kg. The pediatric PN Order provides guidelines for electrolyte requirements per liter for patients greater than 10 kg.

TABLE 7 - PEDIATRIC PN Continued

Component	Supplied As	Amount Required	Comments
Vit B₁₂	Cyanocobalamin	1 mcg is provided in the Pediatric Multi-vitamin Solution.	Important co-enzyme function related to growth, red and white blood cell maturation. Included in multivitamin solution.
Folic Acid		140 mcg is provided in the Pediatric Multivitamin Solution	Important factor in cellular growth, especially in the maturation of red and white blood cells. Included in multivitamin solution.
Multivitamins	Pediatric Multivitamin Solution	2-3 mL/day*	Each 3 mL vial contains: Vitamin A 2300 IU Pantothenic Acid 5 mg Vitamin D 400 IU Vitamin E 7 IU Ascorbic Acid 80 mg Folic Acid 140 mcg Thiamine (B₁) 1.2 mg Cyanocobalamin (B₁₂) 1 mcg Riboflavin (B₂) 1.4 mg Phytonadione (k₁) 200 mcg Niacinamide 17 IU Biotin 20 mcg Pyridoxine 1 mg *Neonates and infants under 1.75 kg: 2 mL/day Infants and children 1.75 - 30 kg: 3 mL/day
Iron	RBC's or Imferon®	2 mg/day	Start at 5 weeks of age. Higher requirement with unreplaced blood loss or chronic iron deficiency. A test dose of Imferon is necessary before instituting therapy.
Phytonadione (Vit K1)	AquaMephyton®	200 mcg are provided in the Pediatric Multivitamins	Important in the production of certain coagulation factors (prothrombin, VII, IX, X). Deficiency and hemorrhagic diathesis may develop rapidly in neonates who are not being fed enterally. Included in multivitamin solution.

TABLE 7 - PEDIATRIC PN Continued

Component	Supplied As	Amount Required	Comments
Trace Elements Less than 10 kg	Zn Cu Mn Cr Se	300.0 mcg/kg/day 20.0 mcg/kg/day 10.0 mcg/kg/day 0.2 mcg/kg/day 0.8 mcg/kg/day	Each 0.3 mL of trace elements mixture contains: 300.0 mcg Zn 20.0 mcg Cu 10.0 mcg Mn 0.2 mcg Cr 0.8 mcg Se
			Each patient (10-30 kg) should receive 0.3 mL/kg/day of the mixture.
Trace Elements 10-30 kg	Zn Cu Mn Cr Se	100.0 mcg/kg/day 20.0 mcg/kg/day 10.0 mcg/kg/day 0.2 mcg/kg/day 0.8 mcg/kg/day	Each 0.1 mL of trace elements mixture contains: 100.0 mcg Zn 20.0 mcg Cu 10.0 mcg Mn 0.2 mcg Cr 0.8 mcg Se
			Each patient (10-30 kg) should receive 0.1 mL/kg/day of the mixture. In patients with weight greater than 30 kg, use adult trace element solution, 1 mL/day. (See Chapt. VIII.)
Heparin		1 IU/mL	Helps prevent platelet thrombi and clots from forming at the catheter tip. Heparin may be deleted from the TPN of neonates and children on ECMO therapy.

TABLE 8
FLUID RECOMMENDATIONS IN NEWBORN INFANTS

	Premature		Full Term
	<1250 g	≥1250 g	
1st day	100	75	60 - 80 mL/kg
2nd day	100-120	75-100	70 - 90 mL/kg
3rd day	*	*	80 - 100 mL/kg
4th day	*	*	100 - 120 mL/kg
5th day and thereafter	*	*	120 - 140 mL/kg*

Fluid requirements may be increased if insensible losses are increased, e.g., very low birth weight (<1 kg), gastroschisis, omphalocele, and phototherapy. Premature neonates with respiratory distress syndrome who are at risk of developing a patent ductus arteriosus (PDA) should be given fluids more cautiously.

* Increase as needed to meet caloric needs.

TABLE 9
DAILY FLUID RECOMMENDATIONS
IN INFANTS AND CHILDREN AGE ONE MONTH OR OLDER

Weight	Fluid
1 - 10 kg	100 mL/kg/day
10 - 20 kg	1000 mL + 50 mL/each kg over 10 kg
≥20 kg	1500 mL + 20 mL/each kg over 20 kg
	May increase gradually up to
	200 mL/kg for peripheral PN

TABLE 10
BLOOD VALUES MONITORED ROUTINELY DURING PARENTERAL NUTRITION

Frequency of Monitoring

At start of therapy and biweekly*	At start of therapy and weekly	As indicated
Na, K, Cl	SGOT, LDH, alkaline	Copper
Creatinine	phosphatase	
Urea	Bilirubin direct/total	Zinc
Glucose	Triglycerides	Iron
Hgb, Hct, WBC,	Magnesium	Ammonia
platelets	Albumin	Osmolarity
	Calcium, phosphorus	pH

*Serum levels should be monitored more frequently in the premature infant.

TABLE 11
POTENTIAL METABOLIC COMPLICATIONS FROM PN
1. **Electrolyte Imbalance**
   a. Hyper/hyponatremia
   b. Hyper/hypokalemia
   c. Hyper/hypochloremia
   d. Hyper/hypocalcemia
   e. Hyper/hypomagnesemia
   f. Hyper/hypophosphatemia
2. **Carbohydrate Administration**
   a. Hyper/hypoglycemia
   b. Hyperosmolarity and associated osmotic diuresis with dehydration, leading to nonketotic hyperglycemic coma.
3. **Protein Administration**
   a. Cholestatic jaundice
   b. Azotemia
4. **Lipid Administration**
   a. Hyperlipidemia
   b. Alteration of pulmonary function
   c. Displacement of albumin-bound bilirubin by plasma free fatty acid
   d. "Overloading syndrome" - characterized by hyperlipemia, fever, lethargy, liver damage, and coagulation disorders. This has been reported in adults but has been recognized rarely in children.
5. **Trace Element Deficiencies**
   a. Zinc deficiency
   b. Copper deficiency
   c. Chromium deficiency
6. **Essential Fatty Acid Deficiency (EFAD)**
   EFAD occurs if lipid emulsions are not used; the major clinical manifestation is a desquamating skin rash.

TABLE 12
CATEGORIZATION OF UMMC COMMERCIAL PEDIATRIC ENTERAL PRODUCTS

I. **Premature Infant Formulas**
   Enfamil Premature
   SMA Premie
   Similac Special Care
   Enfamil Human Milk Fortifier
   Similac "Natural Care" Human Milk Fortifier

II. **Full Term Cows Milk Based Formulas**
   Enfamil
   Similac
   SMA

III. **Soy Protein Isolate Formulas**
   Prosobee
   Isomil
   Nursoy

IV. **Hypoallergenic Protein Hydrolysate Formulas**
   Nutramigen
   Pregestimil

V. **Modified Fat Source Formula**
   Portagen

VI. **Pediatric Formula**
   Pediasure

XIII. ENTERAL NUTRITION

A. Introduction

Nasoenteric or tube enterostomy feedings are indicated in the patient unable to ingest sufficient nutrients normally by mouth. At least a partially functional gastrointestinal tract is necessary for the success of enteral support. The length and functional level of the gastrointestinal tract available will dictate the amount and type of feeding regimen designed and formula selected. Enteral feeding is contraindicated in the presence of peritonitis, intestinal obstruction, paralytic ileus, G.I. hemorrhage, intractable vomiting/diarrhea, repeated pulmonary aspiration, most fistulas, and severe malabsorption syndromes.

The following discussion is a brief introduction to the principles of formula supplements and the management of patients requiring enteral nutrition support. A more detailed explanation of oral supplements and enteral products appears in *The Physicians Handbook of Nutrition Support*. Copies of this manual are located in patient care areas.

B. Nasoenteric Feeding Tubes

1. Characteristics

   The PEN Team recommends the use of silastic pliable nasoenteric feeding tubes for the administration of enteral nutrition. The Dobhoff® feeding tube is available through Central Sterile Supply. These feeding tubes have the following characteristics:

   a. Size 8 or 12 French.
   b. Come with a metal stylet for ease of insertion.
   c. Coated on the lumen and tip with a substance called hydromer. The hydromer becomes slick when wet, allowing for ease of administration of feedings and medications.
   d. Made of soft polyurethane which will not stiffen over time.
   e. The tubes are comfortable and preferable alternatives to the stiff, irritating Salem-Sump-type nasogastric tubes previously used.
   f. These tubes cannot be used for gastric suction or lavage.

C. Placement of Feeding Tube

1. Equipment

   a. Tube and stylet for 8 French tube
   b. Gloves
   c. Water for lubrication of tube
   d. Glass of water and straw, or ice chips
   e. 50 mL luer lock syringe
   f. Emesis basin
   g. Tape

2. Procedure

The insertion technique for small feeding tubes is similar to that of other nasogastric tubes. The patients should be informed of the reason for the placement of the tube and encouraged to facilitate the insertion process (swallowing water or ice chips if able). Staff nurses may place tubes after attending a unit inservice on this topic.

Feeding tubes can be placed in the stomach, duodenum, or jejunum as follows:

a. Stomach: by immediate placement.

1) Position the patient with his head elevated, and measure the distance from the ear, to the tip of the nose, and then to the xyphoid process as the appropriate length of tube needed so that the tip of the tubing is well into the stomach.

2) Irrigate the tube with 10 mL of water, insert the stylet, and lock in place. Lubricate the tip of the tube with water and lubricant as needed.

3) Insert the tube, and confirm the position by aspiration of gastric contents or x-ray with the stylet in place. Remove the stylet only after confirming the position of the tube.

CAUTION: THE STYLET MUST NEVER BE RE-INSERTED WHILE THE TUBE IS IN THE PATIENT. THE STYLET COULD EXIT OUT THE SMALL HOLES AT THE END OF THE TUBE AND PERFORATE THE ESOPHAGEAL OR GASTRIC MUCOSA.

b. Duodenum or jejunum: immediate placement of the tube can be done under fluoroscopy for accurate positioning, or in the stomach with slow advancement into the duodenum or jejunum by peristalsis (after the stylet has been removed). Metoclopramide may be used to increase peristalsis.

1) Tape the tube to the cheek bone with a generous loop; retape as peristalsis moves the tube. Position patient on **right** side to promote passage through the pylorus.

2) An alternative method is to advance the tube one to two inches every two hours, each time irrigating the tube, remarking and taping the loop.

The tube should advance past the pylorus within 24 hours. The position of the tube should be confirmed by abdominal x-ray. Any patient who has aspirated previously, has had problems with gastric retention, nausea and vomiting, or who is disoriented or comatose should have the tube placed beyond the pylorus, even if this requires the use of fluoroscopy. This reduces the possibility of aspiration pneumonia.

D. Care of the Feeding Tube.

Silastic nasoenteric tubes require some special care.

1. Checking for Residual

Because of the small size of the tube, the lumen tends to collapse making it difficult to aspirate stomach contents. To ease the process, the tube should first be irrigated with approximately 10 mL of water. If residual obtained is greater than 100 mL, hold feeding for two hours and remeasure. Aspirated stomach contents should be refed to the patient to prevent loss of fluid and electrolytes.

2. Irrigation

The tube should be irrigated with 10 mL of water every six hours, if the patient is on continuous feedings. If intermittent feedings are provided, 20-50 mL of water should be instilled into the tube after each feeding.

3. Feedings

Very thick feedings or medications need to be diluted before attempting passage down the tube. Irrigation of the tube after the feeding is important to avoid clogging. (Refer to The Physicians Handbook of Nutrition Support for information on enteral product-medication interactions.)

4. General Care

a. Formula should not be hung for longer than four hours.
b. Bag and tubing should be changed every 24 hours.
c. Opened formula should be refrigerated and discarded 24 hours after opening.
d. Whenever possible, continuous drip feedings should be administered via an enteral feeding pump in order to ensure a uniform rate of administration and to decrease complications. Priority for feeding pumps should be given to those patients who are diabetic, on fluid restrictions, who are on continuous feedings through a jejunostomy or who have a history of repeated aspiration.
e. Patients should have their head elevated at least 30° while receiving tube feedings, and this position should be maintained for one hour after the feedings.
f. With each administration, the amount of feeding should be accurately recorded on the patient's Intake and Output sheet. The amount should be separated from other P.O. intake.
g. Tube feedings in patients with a continuous drip infusion who require the head of the bed to be flat for weights, nasotracheal suctioning, or percussion and postural drainage should have their feedings held 30 minutes before treatments.

E. Monitoring Patients on Enteral Nutrition

Patients receiving tube feedings should be monitored according to the following protocol:

1. Daily weights.
2. Accurate intake and output every eight-hour shift.
3. Tube position confirmed by aspiration prior to each feeding or every 6 hours if on continuous feedings.
4. Urine fractionals every eight hours until intake has been stabilized; daily thereafter.
5. Observe during every nursing interaction for evidence of complications: bloating, nausea, diarrhea, dehydration and vomiting.
6. Laboratory tests for hyperglycemia, electrolytes, or changes in renal or hepatic function, daily or weekly as dictated by the patient's underlying disease.

F. Guidelines For Transition From Parenteral To Enteral Nutrition

Inappropriate support of the patient during the transition from parenteral to enteral nutrition frequently occurs when this interval is not clearly planned and monitored. The following guidelines for formula selection and feeding regimen are designed to optimize the reintroduction of enteric support.

1. Formula Selection

   In selecting a formula for any patient, the major factors are caloric density, protein content, osmolality, nutrient complexity, fat content and source and lactose content. The nutrient composition of the enteral products available at the University of Michigan is provided in Appendix F.

   a. **Caloric Density:** All formulas contain between 1-2 kcal/mL. For the transition interval, generally a 1 kcal/mL formula is selected.

   b. **Protein Content and Source:** The enteral formulas stocked at the University of Michigan Hospitals contain 4-22% of their total calories as protein. The most commonly used sources of protein include: soy protein isolates, casein, lactoalbumin, egg albumin, and crystalline amino acids. The protein equivalency of all of these sources is nutritionally comparable; the various sources can be readily interchanged.

   c. **Osmolality:** Osmolality is a measure of the oncotic pressure exerted by a solution. Soluble minerals and carbohydrate primarily determine the osmolality of a formula. An isotonic formula (osmolality ≤350 mOsm/kg water) should be selected for the transition interval whenever possible. If a hypertonic formula is necessary this should initially be diluted. Infusion of hypertonic formula, particularly into small bowel, is often not well tolerated and may lead to diarrhea and cramping.

   d. **Nutrient Complexity:** Some enteral formulas have nutrients in an elemental form. These formulas have minimal residue, low viscosity, are lactose free, and hypertonic. These nutrients are readily absorbable, e.g., mono-and di-saccharides, amino acids, di- and tripeptides, medium chain triglycerides (MCT), and long chain triglycerides. Because of the elemental composition, these formulas do not elicit the same degree of secretory response as the more complex formulas. Feeding elemental formulas during the transition interval results in decreased levels of the digestive enzymes and secretions which are known to stimulate mucosal growth and regeneration. Animal and clinical studies have yet to successfully demonstrate the efficacy of using these products over formulas containing whole protein. The main clinical advantage appears to be in patients with entero-cutaneous fistulas who benefit from the minimal residue and reduced volume of enteric secretions.

   e. **Fat Content and Source:** The formulas stocked at the University of Michigan Hospitals contain a range of fat from 3-36% of the total calories. The primary sources of fat used include corn oil, safflower oil, sunflower oil, and soy oil. There is little documented difference in tolerance to these different fat sources. Some of these products contain a higher percentage of their fat as MCT oil. This is beneficial in patients with diminished sources of lipase.

f. **Lactose Content:** Lactase activity is temporarily lost in many patients during malnutrition due to severe illness and while maintained on TPN. In these instances, a formula with a modified carbohydrate source is indicated. Therefore, it is generally indicated to make the transition from parenteral support with a lactose-free formula. Categorization of the UMH commercial enteral products are provided in Table 13.

2. Feeding Regimen Design

The preferred method of reintroduction of enteral support in the transition interval is via a continous drip over a 24-hour period. The following guidelines for feeding regimen design have been developed for management of this interval.

a. Determine the energy, protein, vitamin, mineral and fluid requirements.
b. Determine the volume of full-strength formula needed to meet these nutritional requirements. To determine the desired hourly volume, divide the total daily volume by the number of hours the patient is to receive the feeding.
c. Initiate feedings of ½ kcal/mL isotonic lactose-free formula at a rate of 40-60 mL hour.
d. Increase the volume by 1.5-2 times the volume infused on day 1 every 12 hours until half the desired hourly volume is tolerated. At this point decrease the TPN support to 50% of its original rate.
e. Continue to increase the volume of feedings gradually as tolerated. When 75% of the desired hourly volume is tolerated, the TPN support is decreased to 25% of its original rate.
f. When the desired hourly volume of feedings is tolerated, the formula concentration is advanced to ¾ strength for 24 hours and finally to full strength. The TPN support is then discontinued. TPN tapering schedule is designed to minimize the amount of TPN wastage.

Table 14 outlines potential complications and preventive interventions for tube feeding administration.

3. Ordering Enteral Nutrition Products

Not all commercially available products are stored at The University of Michigan Hospitals. Many products are similar in composition. Therefore, only one type of formula in each category is available. Appendices F and G provide a list of adult and pediatric products currently available at the hospital.

Products will be delivered to patient areas three times each day: 9:30 a.m., 1:00 p.m. and 6:00 p.m.

Consult the *Physicians Handbook of Nutrition Support*, pp. 35-39, for more information on tube feeding administration.

TABLE 13
CATEGORIZATION OF UMH COMMERCIAL ADULT ENTERAL PRODUCTS

I. NUTRITIONALLY COMPLETE, LACTOSE FREE
   1 kcal/mL
   Standard Protein (<20% of total kcal as protein):
   Ensure, Isocal, Osmolite HN, Precision Isotonic
   Fiber Containing:
   Enrich, Jevity
   Low Fat, Oligomeric:
   Criticare HN
   High Protein (>20% of total kcals as protein):
   Isotein HN

   2 kcal/mL
   Standard Protein:
   Two Cal HN

II. SPECIALIZED FORMULAS
   Hepatic Encephalopathy:
   Travasorb Hepatic
   Renal Failure:
   Amin-Aid
   Respiratory Failure:
   Pulmocare

IV. MODULAR SUPPLEMENTS
   Protein:
   Propac
   Carbohydrate:
   Polycose
   Fat:
   MCT oil, Microlipid
   Carbohydrate & Fat:
   Duocal

V. ORAL SUPPLEMENTS
   Lactose free:
   Ensure, Precision Isotonic, Isotein HN, Two Cal HN, Pulmocare
   Low Residue, Low Fat:
   Citrotein
   High Fiber:
   Enrich
   Milk based:
   Meritene

TABLE 14
POTENTIAL COMPLICATIONS OF TUBE FEEDING AND PREVENTIVE INTERVENTION

Complication	Possible Reasons	Suggested Treatment
GI Disturbances		
Diarrhea	Osmotic overload	Decrease concentration of solution. May require judicious use of anti-diarrheal medications. Continuous feedings rather than bolus.
	Lactose intolerance	Change soluton to lactose-free.
	Contaminated solution or infusion set	Change solution and infusion set. Adhere to standards of clean technique.
	Nervous tension, pain	Promote restful environment.
	Bacterial overgrowth; p.o. medications	Stool culture; review medications and possible side effects.
	Low residue feedings	Use of fiber-enriched formula may be helpful.
Nausea	Volume overload	Decrease total volume/flow rate.
Vomiting	Obstruction; painful or exertional activities immediately after eating	Reassess GI tract function. (UGI series) Allow 45 min rest period after eating.
Cramping Delayed Gastric Emptying	Lactose intolerance	Change to lactose-free formula.
Constipation	Insufficient fluid intake.	Increase fluid intake.
	Decreased bowel motility.	Increase physical activity as tolerated.
	Low residue feedings	Use of fiber-enriched formula may be helpful.

TABLE 14 (Continued)

Complication	Possible Reasons	Suggested Treatment
Dehydration	Insufficient free water administered	Increase fluid intake Administer an additional one-half the total volume of feeding as water when no other free water is given.
Overhydration	Excess fluid administration	Decrease volume of fluid administered.
	Renal, cardiac or pulmonary insufficiency	Monitor electrolytes, decrease sodium intake. Switch to appropriate organ-failure formula.
Aspiration	Rapid administration of feeding	Decrease administration flow rate, monitor residuals.
	Flat position of patient during and after feeding	Raise head of bed 30° during continuous feeding and also for 1 hour after bolus feedings.
	Tube malposition	Confirm placement prior to initiation of feeding and after coughing spells.
	Emesis after feedings	Place tube beyond pylorus as indicated. Schedule exertional activities to avoid feeding times.
Biochemical Imbalance		
Altered Glucose, Altered Electro-lytes, Altered LFT's, and Altered RFT's	Excess or insufficient fluid administration Low Na content in tube feedings or too much free H_2O	Monitor glucose: sudden glucose intolerance may indicate sepsis. Measure electrolytes, I & O. Weigh regularly and adjust feeding solution accordingly.
	Organ system failure	Renal or liver disease may indicate need to decrease protein content of the formula.

TABLE 14 (Continued)

Complication	Possible Reasons	Suggested Treatment
Insufficient Weight Gain	Insufficient calories	Increase concentration and/or volume given.
	Increased metabolic rate	May document with indirect calorimetry (metabolic lab) and increase calories given.
	Malabsorption	Modify feeding content.
Rapid Weight Gain	Excess calories	Decrease calories given.
	Fluid-electrolyte imbalance	Monitor electrolytes, I & O, weight.
Depression, Withdrawal, Non-Compliance	Altered body image	Promote socialization at meal times. Promote mobility. Provide emotional support.
	Loss of oral gratification	Ice chips, sugarfree gum, hard candies if permissible. Provide oral care every shift.
	Lack of information about purpose and duration of enteral therapy	Explain therapy to patient and family. Provide progress reports. Involve patient in care planning and implementation.

XIV. HOME PARENTERAL NUTRITION

Home Parenteral Nutrition (HPN) is available for selected patients at the University of Michigan Hospitals. HPN may be used with those patients requiring short-term as well as long-term parenteral support. Successful HPN requires a strong commitment by the patient and one other family member or close friend who is prepared to act as backup support. Both the patient and the "significant other" must demonstrate a mastery of necessary skills and sterile technique, pharmaceutical compounding and ability to handle aseptically the lines and IV containers prior to being discharged home.

Approximately two weeks are required for HPN inpatient education. Therefore, early initiation of the training is necessary to assure discharge in a timely fashion. Training is done in the hospital and is carried out by members of the Parenteral and Enteral Nutrition Core Team. The time required for teaching varies, depending on the patient's illness and background.

The following criteria, in conjunction with the above conditions, indicate potential HPN candidates:

1. Crohn's Disease
   a. Multiple bowel resection
   b. Severe disease of the remaining gastrointestinal tract

2. Catastrophic Intra-Abdominal Conditions
   a. Radiation enteritis
   b. Fistula or obstruction

3. Short Bowel Syndrome
   a. Mesenteric infarction
   b. Volvulus
   c. Scleroderma
   d. Granulomatous disease

4. Severe Malabsorptive Syndromes

5. Oncology patients who are being actively treated for their disease and who meet the above criteria may be appropriate HPN candidates.

6. Malnourished patients requiring bowel rest or parenteral nutrition prior to surgical procedures or to introduction of oral feedings.

   Please submit a formal referral, and page the PEN Team if you have a potential candidate. Prior to instituting HPN, a thorough evaluation by the PEN Core Team and the patient's physician is necessary.

   All HPN candidates are offered the services of HomeMed, the University of Michigan's Home Infusion program. HomeMed and the Pen Team handle all of the details of insurance verification, patient education, monitoring, and follow-up in cooperation with the patient's physician. The PEN TEAM maintains a 24-hour on-call for all HPN patients.

   For further information on parenteral nutrition or other parenteral therapy please call HomeMed at 936-Home (4663).

XV. APPENDICES

A. Profile For Fat and For Selected Amino Acid and Dextrose Solution Combinations

B. Daily Parenteral Nutrition (PN) Order and Administration Form for Adolescent and Adult Patients for STANDARD FORMULATIONS H-2060413

C. Daily Parenteral Nutrition (PN) Order and Administration Form for Adolescent and Adult Patients for NON-STANDARD FORMULATIONS H-2060401

D. Daily Parenteral Nutrition (PN) Order and Administration Form for Pediatric Patients H-2060425

E. Daily Parenteral Nutrition (PN) Order and Administration Form for Neonatal Patients H-2060395

F. Nutrient Composition of Adult Commercial Enteral Feeding Products Available at the University of Michigan Hospitals

G. Nutrient Composition of Commercial Infant Formulas Available at the University of Michigan Hospitals

H. Tube Feeding Supplements Available at University of Michigan Hospitals

I. Nutrient Composition of Oral Formulas Prepared by the Department of Dietetics at The University of Michigan Hospitals

J. Recommended Dietary Allowances

K. National Center for Health Statistic and Developmental Growth Charts

PROFILE FOR FAT AND FOR SELECTED AMINO ACID AND DEXTROSE SOLUTION COMBINATIONS

FINAL CONCENTRATIONS	AMINOSYN® 2.5%		AMINOSYN® 4.25%		AMINOSYN® 5.0%		AMINOSYN® -RF 2%	
	mOsm/L	Kcal/L	mOsm/L	Kcal/L	mOsm/L	Kcal/L	mOsm/L	Kcal/800mL
Dextrose 5%	503	270	678	340	753	370	—	—
Dextrose 10%	755	440	930	510	1005	540	—	—
Dextrose 15%	1008	610	1183	680	1258	710	—	—
Dextrose 20%	1260	780	1435	850	1510	880	—	—
Dextrose 25%	1500	950	1675	1020	1750	1050	—	—
Dextrose 35%	2018	1290	2193	1360	2268	1390	—	—
Dextrose 43%	—	—	—	—	—	—	1935	1262
Acetate Content (mEq)	43		45*		74		31.5	
Potassium Content (mEq)	2.7		2.7		2.7		1.5	

	mOsm/L	Kcal/500 mL
Fat Emulsion 10%, 500 mL	276**	550
Fat Emulsion 20%, 500 mL	258**	1000

*Also contains 17.5 mEq chloride.
**Figures cited are for Liposyn® II 10% and 20%.

APPENDIX B

THE UNIVERSITY OF MICHIGAN HOSPITALS

DEPARTMENT OF PHARMACY SERVICES
DAILY PARENTERAL NUTRITION (PN)
ORDER AND ADMINISTRATION FORM
FOR **STANDARD** FORMULATIONS

FOR ADOLESCENT AND ADULT PATIENTS

NAME

ADDRESS
(If Outpatient)

LOCATION

REG. NO.

If No Plate, Print Name and Reg. #

* Consult your Parenteral and Enteral Nutrition Manual or the back of this form for the concentration of Amino Acids, Dextrose and other additives in each of the available PN solutions. If none of the standard formulations meet the needs of your patient, order the PN solution on the blank PN order form #H-2060401.
* These standard formulations may not provide adequate amounts of vitamins needed in disease induced deficiencies (e.g., thiamine in chronic alcoholics). When indicated, additional electrolytes, trace elements, and vitamins may be ordered with the standard formulation.
* Send yellow and pink copies to the Pharmacy by 9:00 PM the day before PN solutions are to be administered. Only a 24 hour supply can be ordered.

Type of Solution	PN Sequence Number			Any ingredients requested in the space below will be in addition to those already in the solution designated on the left.
CENTRAL FORMULATIONS				PN Sequence No.
Mixed Amino Acid Formulation				
Mixed Amino Acid Formulation; Low Potassium and Added Sodium				PN Sequence No.
Mixed Amino Acid Cardiac Formulation: No Sodium				
Essential Amino Acid Formulation				PN Sequence No.
PERIPHERAL FORMULATION				
Mixed Amino Acid Peripheral Formulation				
Flow Rate (ml/hr)				

Circle Percentage of Fat Emulsion 500 ml to be Administered Concomitantly 10% 20%	Physician's Signature and Pager Number Dr. #
Desired Number of 500 ml Bottles _____	
Flow Rate _____ ml/hr	Date Time AM PM
Clerk's Initials Unit Date and Time AM PM	Date PN to be administered:

NURSING ADMINISTRATION RECORD

PN Sequence Number	Date Administered	TIME	AM PM	Administered By
PN Sequence Number	Date Administered	TIME	AM PM	Administered By
PN Sequence Number	Date Administered	TIME	AM PM	Administered By
Fat Emulsion 500 ml Administered	Date Administered	TIME	AM PM	Administered By

ME-2060413/332 REV 4/89		University of Michigan Medical Center	**DAILY PN FOR ADOLESCENT AND ADULT PATIENTS - STANDARD**

APPENDIX B (Continued)

Designated below are the contents of each standard parenteral nutrition solution listed on the PN order form. Multivitamin with Biotin, B_{12} and Folic Acid (per protocol) will be added to the first ordered bottle of the day. Trace Elements (per protocol) will be added daily to the first ordered bottle of the day except in the Essential Amino Acid Formulations and when its omission is specifically requested on this order form by the house officer. Check your manual for a detailed content of the multivitamin with Biotin, B_{12} and Folic Acid and trace elements preparations. Regular Human Insulin will be added when ordered by the physician. Phytonadione (Vitamin K₁), 5 mg will be added to the first bottle weekly (Monday) of parenteral nutrition solution. Vitamin K₁ will be omitted when specifically requested on this order form by the house officer.

MIXED AMINO ACID FORMULATION

Amino Acids	(4.25%)	42.5	g
Dextrose	(25%)	250	g
Calcium		4.5	mEq
Magnesium		5	mEq
Potassium		40	mEq
Sodium		35	mEq
Acetate		74.5	mEq
Chloride		52.5	mEq
Phosphorus		12	mM
Heparin Sodium		1000	Units

Volume: 1050 ml   Caloric Value: 1020 Kcal
Approx. Osmolarity: 1825 mOsm

MIXED AMINO ACID FORMULATION: LOW POTASSIUM AND ADDED SODIUM

Amino Acids	(4.25%)	42.5	g
Dextrose	(25%)	250	g
Calcium		4.5	mEq
Magnesium		5	mEq
Potassium		23	mEq
Sodium		51	mEq
Acetate		74.5	mEq
Chloride		52.5	mEq
Phosphorus		12	mM
Heparin Sodium		1000	Units

Volume: 1050 ml   Caloric Value: 1020 Kcal
Approx. Osmolarity: 1825 mOsm

MIXED AMINO ACID CARDIAC FORMULATION: NO SODIUM

Amino Acids	(4.25%)	42.5	g
Dextrose	(35%)	350	g
Calcium		4.5	mEq
Magnesium		8	mEq
Potassium		40	mEq
Acetate		45	mEq
Chloride		37.5	mEq
Gluconate		4.5	mEq
Phosphorus		12	mM
Sulfate		8	mEq
Heparin Sodium		1000	Units

Volume: 1050 ml   Caloric Value: 1360 Kcal
Approx. Osmolarity: 2325 mOsm

MIXED AMINO ACID **PERIPHERAL** FORMULATION

Amino Acids	(2.5%)	25	g
Dextrose	(10%)	100	g
Calcium		4.5	mEq
Magnesium		5	mEq
Potassium		23	mEq
Sodium		47	mEq
Acetate		72.5	mEq
Chloride		35	mEq
Phosphorus		9	mM
Heparin Sodium		1000	Units

Volume: 1050 ml   Caloric Value: 440 Kcal
Approx. Osmolarity: 880 mOsm
To be infused with Fat Emulsion

ESSENTIAL AMINO ACID FORMULATION

Essential Amino Acids	(2%)	15.7	g
Dextrose	(43%)	350	g
Potassium		1.5	mEq
Acetate		31.5	mEq
Heparin Sodium		1000	Units

Volume: 800 ml   Caloric Value: 1253 Kcal
Approx. Osmolarity: 1935 mOsm

Physicians may request additions to the standard PN solution - but only phosphate salts (potassium or sodium) may be deleted. When reduction of other electrolytes is deemed necessary, physicians must write the detailed order on the DAILY PN FOR ADOLESCENT AND ADULT PATIENTS - NONSTANDARD, FORM H-2060401.

APPENDIX C

THE UNIVERSITY OF MICHIGAN HOSPITALS
DEPARTMENT OF PHARMACY SERVICES
DAILY PARENTERAL NUTRITION (PN)
ORDER AND ADMINISTRATION FORM
FOR **NON-STANDARD** FORMULATIONS
FOR ADOLESCENT AND ADULT PATIENTS

NAME

ADDRESS
(If Outpatient)

LOCATION

REG. NO.

If No Plate, Print Name and Reg. #

For patients weighing 30kg. or more. Only a 24 hour supply can be ordered.
Use this form to order Parenteral Nutrition solutions ONLY when none of the standard formulations listed on Form #H-2060413 meet the needs of your patient. Send yellow and pink copies to Pharmacy by 9:00 P.M. the day before PN solutions are to be administered.

BASE SOLUTION	PN Sequence Number	PN Sequence Number	PN Sequence Number
Final Concentration of Crystalline Amino Acid in Solution _____ %	Total Volume of PN Solution Ordered	Total Volume of PN Solution Ordered	Total Volume of PN Solution Ordered
Final Concentration of Special Amino Acid. Specify _____ %			
Final Concentration of Dextrose in Solution _____ %	ml	ml	ml

ADDITIVES	SEE THE BACK OF THIS FORM FOR IMPORTANT INFORMATION		
Calcium Gluconate	mEq	mEq	mEq
Magnesium Sulfate	mEq	mEq	mEq
Potassium Acetate	mEq	mEq	mEq
Potassium Chloride	mEq	mEq	mEq
Potassium Phosphate	mM	mM	mM
Sodium Acetate	mEq	mEq	mEq
Sodium Chloride	mEq	mEq	mEq
Sodium Phosphate	mM	mM	mM
Multivitamin with Biotin B_{12} and Folic Acid	☐ Yes Per Protocol ☐ No	☐ Yes Per Protocol ☐ No	☐ Yes Per Protocol ☐ No
Trace Elements	☐ Yes Per Protocol ☐ No	☐ Yes Per Protocol ☐ No	☐ Yes Per Protocol ☐ No
Heparin Sodium	☐ Yes Per Protocol ☐ No	☐ Yes Per Protocol ☐ No	☐ Yes Per Protocol ☐ No
Regular Human Insulin	units	units	units
Flow Rate (ml/hr)			

Circle Percentage of Fat Emulsion To Be Administered Concomitantly   10%   20%

Desired Number of 500 ml Bottles _____
Flow Rate _____ ml/hr

Clerk's Initials	Unit	Date	and	Time	
					AM PM

Physician's Signature   and   Pager Number   Dr. #

Date   Time   AM PM

Date PN To Be Administered _____

NURSING ADMINISTRATION RECORD

PN Sequence Number	Date Administered	Time	AM PM	Administered By
PN Sequence Number	Date Administered	Time	AM PM	Administered By
PN Sequence Number	Date Administered	Time	AM PM	Administered By
Fat Emulsion 500 ml Administered	Date Administered	Time	AM PM	Administered By

ME-2060401/331 Rev. 4/89

University of Michigan Medical Center

DAILY PN FOR ADOLESCENT AND ADULT PATIENTS-NON STANDARD

APPENDIX C (Continued)

Use this form to order Parenteral Nutrition for adolescent and adult patients weighing 30kg or more. Consult your Parenteral and Enteral Nutrition Manual for the safe and effective use of all PN ingredients. The following are guidelines for ordering PN solutions.

1. Base Solution:

Type of Patient	Total Volume of PN solution to be ordered per bottle	Final concentration of crystalline amino acid solution	Final concentration of essential amino acid solution	Final concentration of Dextrose solution
normal liver and renal function	1,000 ml	4.25% (1)		25% (Central infusion)
chronic or acute renal failure	800 ml		2% (2)	43% (Central infusion)
or	1,000 ml	2.5 % (3)		35% (Central infusion)
liver dysfunction	1,000 ml	2.5 % (3)		25% (Central infusion)
cardiac pt. with fluid restrictions	1,000 ml	4.25% (1)		35% (Central infusion)
peripheral supplementation for pts. with normal renal & liver function	1,000 ml	2.5 % (3)		10% (Peripheral infusion)

These solutions provide electrolytes in the amounts listed below. Any electrolytes requested on this form will be in addition to those already in the solution:

(1) provides 45 mEq acetate, 17.5 mEq chloride, and 2.7 mEq potassium.
(2) provides 31.5 mEq acetate and 1.5 mEq potassium.
(3) provides 43 mEq acetate and 2.7 mEq potassium.

2. Additives:

a. Electrolytes

Electrolytes	Recommended Daily Requirement		Compatibility Per Liter of Solution
Calcium	10-15 mEq/day	(5 mEq/l)	(up to) 10 mEq
Magnesium	8-24 mEq/day	(8 mEq/l)	(up to) 12 mEq
Potassium	90-240 mEq/day	(20-50 mEq/l)	(up to) 80 mEq
Sodium	60-150 mEq/day	(20-50 mEq/l)	Wide Range
Acetate	80-120 mEq/day	(30-50 mEq/l)	Wide Range
Chloride	60-150 mEq/day	(20-50 mEq/l)	Wide Range
Phosphorus*	30-50 mM/day	(10-15 mM/l)	(up to) 20 mM

*1 mM Potassium phosphate provides 1.47 mEq Potassium.
1 mM Sodium phosphate provides 1.33 mEq Sodium.

b. Vitamins added per protocol:

The following vitamins are provided per protocol, daily, as follows:

1) Multivitamin with Biotin, B_{12} and Folic Acid, 10 ml in the first bottle of the day provide the following vitamins:

Ascorbic Acid	100	mg	Pyridoxine HCl (B_6)	4 mg	Biotin		60 mcg
Vitamin A	3,300	IU	Niacinamide	40 mg	Vitamin B_{12}		5 mcg
Vitamin D	200	IU	Dexpanthenol	15 mg	Folic Acid		400 mcg
Thiamine HCl (B_1)	3	mg	Vitamin E	10 IU			
Riboflavin (B_2)	3.6	mg					

2.) Phytonadione-Vitamin K_1, 5 mg should be administered in the parenteral nutrition solution weekly (Monday), except when the patient is on anti-coagulation therapy.

c. Trace Elements added per protocol:

1 ml will be provided, per protocol in one bottle once a day. Patients with chronic and acute renal failure, and those with liver dysfunction may require adjusting this schedule.

1 ml of trace elements provides:

Zinc	5 mg	Manganese	0.5 mg	Selenium	0.04 mg
Copper	1 mg	Chromium	0.01 mg		

d. Heparin added per protocol:

1,000 units will be provided, per protocol with each 1,000 ml of PN solution.

e. Regular Human Insulin:

To be administered only as indicated by persistent elevation of blood glucose.

3. Fat Emulsion:

Unless contraindicated, up to 60% of daily caloric intake can be supplemented as fat. Recommended daily dosage is 1-3 g/kg/day.

APPENDIX D

THE UNIVERSITY OF MICHIGAN HOSPITALS

DEPARTMENT OF PHARMACY SERVICES

DAILY PARENTERAL NUTRITION (PN)

ORDER AND ADMINISTRATION FORM

FOR PEDIATRIC PATIENTS

NAME

ADDRESS
(If Outpatient)

LOCATION

REG. NO.

If No Plate, Print Name and Reg. #

For patients weighing 10-30 kg.
Send yellow and pink copies to Mott Pharmacy by 9:00 P.M. the day before the PN solution is to be administered. Pharmacy will then deliver by 8:00 A.M. C
a 24 hour supply can be ordered.

STANDARD CENTRAL FORMULATION		STANDARD PERIPHERAL FORMULATION		NON-STANDARD FORMULATION		
PN Sequence Number		PN Sequence Number		PN Sequence Number		
Total Volume of PN Solution Ordered	ml	Total Volume of PN Solution Ordered	ml	Total Volume of PN Solution Ordered		
Flow Rate	ml/hr	Flow Rate	ml/hr	Flow Rate		m
Patient's Weight	kg	Patient's Weight	kg	Patient's Weight		
CONTENT PER 1000 ml		CONTENT PER 1000 ml				
Amino Acids (3.5%)	35 g	Amino Acids (2.0%)	20 g	Final Concentration of Crystalline Amino Acid Solution	g	
Dextrose (25%)	250 g	Dextrose (10%)	100 g	Final Concentration of Special Amino Acids, Specify	g	
Calcium	9 mEq	Calcium	9 mEq	Final Concentration of Dextrose in Solution	%	
Magnesium	5 mEq	Magnesium	5 mEq	Calcium Gluconate	mEq	
Potassium	40 mEq	Potassium	30 mEq	Magnesium Sulfate	mEq	
Sodium	35 mEq	Sodium	35 mEq	Potassium Acetate	mEq	
Acetate	82 mEq	Acetate	60 mEq	Potassium Chloride	mEq	
Chloride	35 mEq	Chloride	35 mEq	Potassium Phosphate	mM	
Phosphorus	12 mM	Phosphorus	6 mM	Sodium Acetate	mEq	
Pediatric Multivitamin ☐ Yes ☐ No Per Protocol		Pediatric Multivitamin ☐ Yes ☐ No Per Protocol		Sodium Chloride	mEq	
Pediatric Trace Elements ☐ Yes ☐ No Per Protocol		Pediatric Trace Elements ☐ Yes ☐ No Per Protocol		Sodium Phosphate	mM	
Heparin ☐ Yes ☐ No Per Protocol		Heparin ☐ Yes ☐ No Per Protocol		Pediatric Multivitamin	☐ Yes ☐ No Per Protocol	
Provides 990 Kcal		Provides 420 Kcal		Pediatric Trace Elements	☐ Yes ☐ No Per Protocol	
Any ingredients requested in the space below will be in addition to those already in the solution designated above.				Heparin	☐ Yes ☐ No Per Protocol	
Additive(s) per 1000 ml:				Parenteral Iron	mg	

Circle Percentage of Fat Emulsion To Be Administered Concomitantly   10%   20%

Volume Ordered _____ ml

Flow Rate _____ ml/hr

Clerk's Initials   Unit   Date   and   Time
AM
PM

Physician's Signature   and   Pager Number   Dr. #

Date   Time   AM PM

Date PN to be Administered _____

NURSING ADMINISTRATION RECORD

PN Sequence Number	Date Administered	Time	AM PM	Administered By
PN Sequence Number	Date Administered	Time	AM PM	Administered By
Fat Emulsion 500 ml Administered	Date Administered	Time	AM PM	Administered By

ME-2060425/333
REV. 4/89

University of Michigan Medical Center

DAILY PN FOR PEDIATRIC PATIENT

APPENDIX D (Continued)

Use this form to order parenteral nutrition for pediatric patients weighing 10-30 kg. For patients weighing over 30 kg, please use Form H-2060401: DAILY PARENTERAL NUTRITION (PN) ORDER AND ADMINISTRATION FORM FOR NON-STANDARD FORMULATIONS FOR ADOLESCENT AND ADULT PATIENTS, or Form H-2060413 FOR STANDARD FORMULATIONS. For patients under 10 kg, use the Daily PN for Neonatal Patients, Form H-2060395.

Consult the Chapter on Pediatric Nutrition (Chapter XII), of the Parenteral and Enteral Nutrition Manual, for the safe and effective use of all parenteral nutrition (PN) ingredients. The following are guidelines for ordering PN solutions:

A. Standard Pediatric PN Solutions:

The two standard solutions available from Mott Pharmacy are for:

  a. Central Administration   b. Peripheral Administration

The content of each standard formulation is listed on the front of the form. These formulations provide maintenance requirements for patients over 5 kg. Physicians may request additions to the standard PN solutions but not deletions. When deletion of certain electrolytes or vitamins are indicated, an individualized non-standard order should be written on this same form. Vitamins and heparin are automatically added. Trace elements should be requested daily according to patient's weight.

B. Individualized Non-standard Pediatric PN Solutions:

1. Base Solution:

Weight	Maintenance Fluid Requirement ml/kg/24 hours	Final Concentration of Crystalline Amino Acid Solution Peripheral	Central	Final Concentration of Dextrose Solution (Peripheral Infusion)	Final Concentration of Dextrose Solution (Central Infusion)
10-20 kg	1000 ml + 50 ml/kg over 10 kg	2.0%	3.5%	10%	25%
20-30 kg	1500 ml + 20 ml/kg over 20 kg	2.0%	3.5%	10%	25%

Parenteral nutrition volumes should be ordered in multiples of 100 ml to last 24 hours.

2. Additives:

a. Electrolytes

	Recommended Daily Requirement	Compatibility Per Liter of Solution
Calcium	5-20 mEq/day (9 mEq/l)	(up to) 10 mEq
Magnesium	4-24 mEq/day (5 mEq/l)	(up to) 12 mEq
Potassium	20-240 mEq/day (20-50 mEq/l)	(up to) 80 mEq
Sodium	20-150 mEq/day (20-50 mEq/l)	wide Range
Acetate	20-120 mEq/day (30-50 mEq/l)	wide Range
Chloride	20-150 mEq/day (20-50 mEq/l)	wide Range
Phosphate*	6-50 mM/day (5-15 mM/l)	(up to) 20 mM

Calcium - Phosphate Precipitation Factor

$$\frac{[(\text{Calcium mEq}) + (\text{Phosphate mM})] \times 1000}{\text{Total Infusion Volume per Bottle}} \leq 30$$

Adjust Calcium or Phosphate to maintain Precipitation Factor ≤ 30 (per 1000 ml).

  * 1 mM Potassium phosphate provides 1.47 mEq potassium.
    1 mM Sodium phosphate provides 1.33 mEq sodium.

b. Vitamins provided per protocol:

Pediatric Multivitamin Injection (one vial/day) — one vial diluted to 3 ml.

One vial of pediatric multivitamin injection contains:

Ascorbic Acid	80	mg	Pyridoxine (B_6)	1	mg	Cyanocobalamin (B_{12})	1 mcg
Vitamin A	2300	IU	Niacinamide	17	mg	Phytonadione (K_1)	200 mcg
Vitamin D	400	IU	Dexpanthenol	5	mg	Biotin	20 mcg
Thiamine (B_1)	1.2	mg	Vitamin E	7	IU		
Riboflavin (B_2)	1.4	mg	Folic Acid	140	mcg		

c. Pediatric Trace Elements Formulation provided per protocol:
  0.1 ml of this formulation provides:

Zinc	100 mcg	Copper	20 mcg	Selenium	0.8 mcg
Manganese	10 mcg	Chromium	0.2 mcg		

d. Parenteral Iron: Contact PEN Team for dosing and additional information.

e. Heparin provided per protocol:

f. Regular Human Insulin: To be administered only as indicated by persistent elevation of blood glucose above 250 mg/dl.

3. Fat Emulsion 10% and 20%:
  Unless contraindicated, up to 50% of daily caloric intake can be supplied as fat.
  Recommended dosage 1-4 g/kg/day
  Fat Emulsion 10% provides 1.1 Kcal/ml
  Fat Emulsion 20% provides 2.0 Kcal/ml

APPENDIX E

THE UNIVERSITY OF MICHIGAN HOSPITALS

DEPARTMENT OF PHARMACY SERVICES
DAILY PARENTERAL NUTRITION (PN)
ORDER AND ADMINISTRATION FORM
FOR NEONATAL PATIENTS

NAME

ADDRESS
(If Outpatient)

LOCATION

REG. NO.

If No Plate, Print Name and Reg. #

For Patients weighing less than 10 kg.

Send yellow and pink copies to Mott Pharmacy by 9:00 P.M. the day before the PN solution is to be administered. Pharmacy will then deliver by 8:00 A.M. the day the solution is to be administered. Only a 24 hour supply can be ordered.

BASE SOLUTION AND ADDITIVES	
PN Sequence Number	
Patient's Weight	kg
Infusion Volume of PN Solution Ordered/Kg	ml/kg
Total Infusion Volume of PN Solution Ordered	ml
Flow Rate	ml/hr
Crystalline Amino Acid Solution	g/kg
Final Concentration of Dextrose in Solution	%
Calcium Gluconate	mEq/kg
Phosphate (See back)	mM/kg
Precipitation Factor (Formula on reverse side)	/100ml
Magnesium Sulfate	mEq/kg
Potassium	mEq/kg
Sodium	mEq/kg
Pediatric Multivitamin (See back)	Per Protocol
Neonatal Trace Elements (0.3 ml/kg)	Per Protocol
Heparin (0.5 U/ml)	Per Protocol

Circle Percentage of Fat Emulsion to be Administered Concomitantly   10%   20%

Volume Ordered _____ ml

Flow Rate _____ ml/hr

Clerk's Signature (Nurse in Holden)   Unit   Date   and   Time   AM   PM

Physician's Signature   and   Page Number

Date   Time   AM   PM

Date PN to be administered _____

CALORIC PROFILE

Dextrose: (%) (ml infused vol) (0.034) =	Kcal Dextrose
Fat Emulsion: 10% = 1.1 Kcal/ml, 20% = 2 Kcal/ml (ml infused vol) (Kcal/ml) =	Kcal Fat Emulsion
Nonprotein Kcal/Kg: [(Kcal Dextrose) + (Kcal Fat)] ÷ (kg) =	Nonprotein Kcal/
Protein: (g infused) (4 Kcal/g) =	Kcal Protein
Total Kcal/Kg: [(Kcal Dextrose) + (Kcal Fat) + (Kcal Protein)] ÷ (kg) =	Total Kcal/kg

NURSING ADMINISTRATION RECORD

PN Sequence Number	Date Administered	Time	AM PM	Administered By
Fat Emulsion Administered	Date Administered	Time	AM PM	Administered By

ME 2060395/457   Rev 4/89

University of Michigan Medical Center

DAILY PN FOR NEONATAL PATIENTS

88

APPENDIX E (Continued)

Use this form to order parenteral nutrition (PN) for neonatal patients weighing less than 10 kg. For patients weighing over 10 kg, please use Form H-2060425 DAILY PARENTERAL NUTRITION (PN) ORDER AND ADMINISTRATION FORM FOR PEDIATRIC PATIENTS.

Consult the chapter on Pediatric Nutrition (Chapter XII), of the Parenteral and Enteral Nutrition Manual, for the safe and effective use of all PN ingredients. The following are guidelines for ordering PN solutions:

1. BASE SOLUTION: Use the table below to estimate volumes to infuse. Overfill will automatically be provided by Pharmacy.

A. Fluids:

	ESTIMATED MAINTENANCE *ml/kg/24 hr			
DAY	PREMATURE		FULL TERM	
	<1250g	>1250g		*Patients under radiant warmers or receiving phototherapy may require an additional 15-25 ml/kg/24 hr.
1	100	75	60-75	
2	100-120	75-100	75-85	
3	Increase as tolerated to meet caloric needs.			

B. Protein:

Suggested Nonprotein Calorie and Protein combinations to maximize protein utilization:

Protein g/kg/24 hr	Nonprotein Calories Kcal/kg/24 hr
1	25
2	50
2.5	70+

C. Dextrose:

Peripheral Concentrations are available in 0.5% increments up to 12.5% (12.5 g/100ml).

Central Formulation: Available in concentrations up to 35%.

Use 4-8 mg/kg/min as a baseline glucose infusion rate; increase as tolerated to provide adequate calories.

2. Fat Emulsion 10% and 20%:

Unless contraindicated, up to 50% of daily caloric intake can be supplied as fat.
Recommended dosage 1-4 g/kg/day (limit to <3g/kg/day in infants with respiratory diseases).
Fat Emulsion 10% provides 1.1 Kcal/ml.
Fat Emulsion 20% provides 2.0 Kcal/ml.

3. Additives:

A. Electrolytes:

	Recommended Daily Requirement
Calcium	0.5-3 mEq/kg
Magnesium	0.5-1 mEq/kg
Potassium	2.0-4 mEq/kg
Sodium	2.0-4 mEq/kg
Phosphate	1.0-1.5 mM/kg

a. Phosphate provided as salt of potassium or sodium. Sodium or potassium used will be subtracted from sodium and/or potassium ordered. Remainder of sodium and/or potassium will be added as chloride salt.

b. Acetate is available if needed. To order, write "Acetate" and the mEq/kg desired in the blank space provided. The salt should not be specified as it will be selected based on the sodium or potassium ordered above.

c. Electrolytes should be ordered in whole or half (0.5) units only.

Calcium-Phosphate Precipitation Factor	$\frac{[(Calcium\ mEq/kg)\ +\ (Phosphate\ mM/kg)]\ x\ Wt(kg)\ x\ 100}{Total\ Infusion\ Volume\ per\ Bottle} \leq 3$	Adjust Calcium or Phosphate to maintain Precipitation Factor ≤ 3 (per 100ml).

B. Vitamins provided per protocol: 1 vial if weight of patient> 1750g, .65 vial if weight of patient < 1750g.

Pediatric Multivitamin Injection (one vial/day)—one vial diluted to 3 ml.

One vial of pediatric multivitamin injection contains:

Ascorbic Acid	80 mg	Pyridoxine (B$_6$)	1 mg	Cyanocobalamin (B$_{12}$)	1 mcg
Vitamin A	2300 IU	Niacinamide	17 mg	Phytonadione (K$_1$)	200 mcg
Vitamin D	400 IU	Dexpanthenol	5 mg	Biotin	20 mcg
Thiamine (B$_1$)	1.2 mg	Vitamin E	7 IU		
Riboflavin (B$_2$)	1.4 mg	Folic Acid	140 mcg		

C. Neonatal Trace Elements Formulation provided per protocol: 0.3 ml/kg/day.
0.3 ml of this formulation provides:

Zinc	300 mcg	Copper	20 mcg	Selenium	0.8 mcg
Manganese	10 mcg	Chromium	0.2 mcg		

D. Heparin provided per protocol: 0.5 U/ml.

E. Parenteral Iron: Contact PEN Team for dosing and additional information.

F. Regular Human Insulin: To be administered only as indicated by persistent elevation of blood glucose above 250 mg/dl.

APPENDIX F
NUTRIENT COMPOSITION OF COMMERCIAL ENTERAL FEEDING PRODUCTS

	LACTOSE FREE		
	Ensure	**Isocal**	**Osmolite HN**
kcal/mL	1.06	1.06	1.06
PROTEIN, gm/L	37.2	32.5	44.4
Source	Sodium and calcium caseinates, soy protein isolate	Calcium and sodium caseinate, soy protein isolate	Sodium and calcium caseinates, soy protein isolate
FAT, gm/L	37.2	42	36.8
Source	Corn oil	Soy oil, MCT oil	Medium chain triglycerides, corn oil, soy oil
CARBOHYDRATE, gm/L	145	126	141
Source	Hydrolyzed corn starch, sucrose	Maltodextrin	Hydrolyzed corn starch
Free water, mL/L	843	843	829
VITAMINS/L:			
Vitamin A, IU/RE	2642/793	2500/750.75	3804/1142
Vitamin D, IU	211	200	304
Vitamin E, IU/TE	31.7/31.7	38/38	34.2/34.2
Vitamin C, mg	161	150	139
Folic Acid, mcg	423	200	465
Thiamine, mg	1.6	1.9	1.7
Riboflavin, mg	1.6	2.2	1.9
Niacin, mg	21.1	25	22.8
Vitamin B$_6$, mg	2.1	2.5	2.3
Vitamin B$_{12}$, mcg	6.3	7.5	7.2
Biotin, mcg	320	150	350
Pantothenic acid, mg	10.6	12.5	11.4
Vitamn K$_1$, mcg	38	125	55
Choline, mcg	320	250	590
MINERALS/L:			
Calcium, mg	528	600	760
Phosphorus, mg	528	500	760
Magnesium, mg	211	200	304
Iron, mg	9.5	9	13.9
Sodium, mg(mEq)	845 (36.7)	500 (21.7)	930 (40.4)
Potassium, mg(mEq)	1564 (40.1)	1000 (32.0)	1564 (40.1)
Chloride, mg	1437	1000	1437
Iodine, mcg	80	75	114
Zinc, mg	11.9	10	17.3
Copper, mg	1.1	1	1.52
Manganese, mg	2.1	2.5	3.8
Volume required to meet 100% RDA, mL	2000	1892	1320
Non-protein kcal:gm nitrogen	154:1	170:1	126:1
mOsm/kg Water	470	300	310
Comments	Oral supplement, gastric feedings.	Not palatable as supplement; gastric and small bowel feedings.	Not palatable; gastric and small bowel feedings.

APPENDIX F (Continued)

	Precision Isotonic	Lactose Free with Fiber: Enrich	Jevity
kcal/mL	0.96	1.10	1.06
PROTEIN, g/L	28.8	39.7	44.5
Source	Egg albumin sodium caseinate	Sodium and calcium caseinates, soy protein isolate	Sodium and calcium caseinates
FAT, g/L	30.1	37.2	36.8
Source	Soybean oil mono- and diglycerides	Corn oil	MCT oil, corn oil
CARBOHYDRATE, gm/L	144.2	161.8	152.2
Source	Maltodextrin, sucrose	Hydrolyzed corn starch, sucrose, 13.9 g soy fiber	Hydrolyzed cornstarch soy fiber 14.3 g soy fiber
Lactose,g/L	0	0	0
Free water, mL/L	923	816	835
VITAMINS/L:			
Vitamin A, IU/RE	3210/962	3804/1142	3786
Vitamin D, IU	256	304	305
Vitamin E, IU/TE	19.2/19.2	34.2/34.2	34.3
Vitamin C, mg	57.7	139	227.2
Folic Acid, mcg	260	465	457.9
Thiamine, mg	1.4	1.9	1.73
Riboflavin, mg	1.7	1.7	1.95
Niacin, mg	12.8	1.9	22.7
Vitamin B_6, mg	1.9	22.8	2.28
Vitamin B_{12}, mcg	3.9	2.3	7.2
Biotin, mcg	190	350	343.4
Pantothenic acid, mg	6.41	11.4	11.36
Vitamin K, mcg	64.1	55	55.1
Choline, mg	64.1	590	454
MINERALS/L:			
Calcium, mg	640	720	912
Phosphorus, mg	640	720	759
Magnesium, mg	256	287	303
Iron, mg	11.5	13.1	13.6
Sodium, mg(mEq)	770 (33.5)	850 (37)	932
Potassium, mg(mEq)	960 (24.6)	1560 (40)	1569
Chloride, mg	1030	1440	1442
Iodine, mcg	96.2	110	113
Zinc, mg	9.6	16.1	17
Copper, mg	1.28	1.44	1.53
Manganese, mg	2.56	3.51	3.77
Volume required to to meet 100• RDA, mL	1560	1530	1320
Non-protein kcal:gm nitrogen	184:1	155:1	116:1
mOsm/kg Water	300	480	310
Comments	Oral supplement; gastric and small bowel feedings.	Oral supplement; gastric and small bowel feedings.	Not palatable; as supplement; gastric and small bowel feedings.

APPENDIX F (Continued)

	Lactose Free High Protein: Isotein HN	Lactose Free High Calorie Two Cal HN	Low Fat, Oligomeric: Criticare HN
kcal/mL	1.2	2.06	1.06
PROTEIN, gm/L	68	84	38
Source	Egg albumin sodium caseinate	Sodium and calcium caseinates, soy protein	Free amino acids, hydrolyzed casein
FAT, g/L	34	89	3
Source	Soybean oil medium chain triglycerides, mono and diglycerides	Corn oil, MCT oil	Safflower oil
CARBOHYDRATE, g/L	156	216	222
Source	Maltodextrin, fructose	Hydrolyzed corn starch, sucrose	Maltodextrin
Lactose, gm/L	0	0	0
Free water, mL/L	847	690	831
VITAMINS/L:			
Vitamin A, IU/RE	2820/847	5263/1580	2600/780.8
Vitamin D, IU	226	421.0	210
Vitamin E, IU/TE	17/17	48/48	40/40
Vitamin C, mg	51	189.5	159
Folic Acid, mcg	230	700	210
Thiamine, mg	1.3	2.5	2
Riboflavin, mg	1.5	2.9	2.2
Niacin, mg	11.3	33.6	26
Vitamin B_6, mg	1.7	3.4	2.6
Vitamin B_{12}, mcg	3.4	10.1	7.9
Biotin, mcg	170	510	159
Pantothenic acid, mg	5.7	16.8	13.2
Vitamin K, mcg	57	75.8	132
Choline, mg	57	800	260
MINERALS/L:			
Calcium, mg	560	1060	530
Phosphorus, mg	560	1060	530
Magnesium, mg	226	421	210
Iron, mg	10.2	18.9	9.5
Sodium, mg(mEq)	680 (29.6)	1052.6 (45.76)	630 (27.4)
Potassium, mg(mEq)	850 (22.8)	2316.0 (59.4)	1320 (33.8)
Chloride, gm	900	1558.0	1060
Iodine, mcg	85	160.0	79
Zinc, mg	8.5	24.0	10
Copper, mg	1.1	1.1	1
Manganese, mg	2.3	6.3	2.6
Volume required to meet 100• RDA, mL	1770	950	1892
Non-protein kcal:gm nitrogen	86:1	125:1	150:1
mOsm/kg Water	300	700	650
Comments	Oral supplement; gastric and small bowel feedings.	Oral supplement; gastric feedings.	Not palatable as oral supplement; gastric feedings.

APPENDIX F (Continued)

	Amin Aid	Travasorb Hepatic	Pulmocare
kcal/mL	2.0	1.1	1.5
PROTEIN, gm/L	19.4	28.6	62.6
Source	Purified crystalline amino acids	Crystalline L-amino acid hydrolyzed casein	Sodium and calcium caseinates
FAT, gm/L	46.2	14.3	92.1
Source	Partially hydrogenated soy bean oil, lecithin, mono and diglycerides	MCT oil, sunflower oil	Corn oil
CARBOHYDRATE, gm/L	365.6	209	105
Source	Maltodextrins oligosaccharide	Glucose oligosaccharide	Hydrolized corn starch, sucrose
Lactose,gm/L	0	0	0
Free water, mL/L	—	770	770
VITAMINS/L:			
Vitamin A, IU/RE	0	1590/477.6	5200/1576
Vitamin D, IU	0	191.6	416
Vitamin E, IU/TE	0	4.9/4.9	47/47
Vitamin C, mg	0	42.9	312
Folic Acid, mcg	0	191.6	832
Thiamine, mg	0	0.7	3.12
Riboflavin, mg	0	0.8	3.5
Niacin, mg	0	8.6	41.6
Vitamin B_6, mg	0	1.1	4.16
Vitamin B_{12}, mcg	0	1.4	12.48
Biotin, mcg	0	25.0	624
Pantothenic acid, mg	0	2.6	20.8
Vitamin K_1, mcg	0	50.1	74.9
Choline, mg	0	191.6	624
MINERALS/L:			
Calcium, mg	0	381	1040
Phosphorus, mg	0	472	1040
Magnesium, mg	0	186	416
Iron, mg	0	9	18.7
Sodium, mg(mEq)	345 (15.0)	435 (18.9)	1289/56
Potassium, mg(mEq)	234 (6.0)	1131 (29.0)	1872/48
Chloride, mg	0	678	1664
Iodine, mcg	0	72	156
Zinc, mg	0	7	23
Copper, mg	0	952	2.08
Manganese, mg	0	1.1	5.2
Volume required to meet 100% RDA, mL	No vitamins or minerals	2268	947
Non-protein kcal: gm nitrogen		211:1	125:1
mOsm/kg Water	1095	690	490
Comments	Oral supplement; gastric feedings.	Oral supplement; gastric and small bowel tube feedings.	Gastric and small bowel tube feeding.

NUTRIENT COMPOSITION OF COMMERCIAL INFANT FORMULAS

Premature Infant Formulas

Nutrient/liter	Enfamil Premature 20	Enfamil Premature 24	Similac Special Care-24	Enfamil Human Milk Fortifier (0.95 g/packet) Per 4 Packets
kcal/mL	0.67	0.8	0.8	14
Protein (g) (% total calories)	20 (12)	24 (12)	22 (11)	.7 (20)
Source	whey/casein 60:40	whey/casein 60:40	whey/casein 60:40	whey/casein 60:40
Fat (g) (% total calories)	34 (45)	40 (45)	44 (48)	.05 (3)
Source	40% MCT 40% corn oil 20% coconut oil	40% MCT 40% corn oil 20% coconut oil	50% 30% soy oil 20% coconut oil	
Carbohydrate (g) (% total of calories)	74 (43)	87 (43)	86 (41)	2.7 (77)
Source	corn syrup solids, and lactose	corn syrup solids, and lactose	hydrolyzed cornstarch lactose	corn syrup solids
Water (g)	891	880	890	
Mineral				
Calcium (mg) (mEq)	1105 (55)	1320 (66)	1460 (73)	60 (3)
Phosphorus (mg)	558	667	730	33
Sodium (mg) (mEq)	262 (11)	310 (14)	350 (15)	7 (.3)
Potassium (mg) (mEq)	745 (19)	880 (23)	1050 (27)	16 (.4)
Chloride (mg) (mEq)	567 (16)	670 (19)	660 (19)	18 (.5)
Magnesium (mg) (mEq)	33 (2.8)	39 (3.3)	100 (8.2)	0
Iron (mg)	1.7	1.9	3	0
Zinc (mg)	6.7	7.9	12	.31
Copper (mg)	1.07	1.26	2.03	.08
Manganese (mg)	0.9	0.1	0.1	.009
Iodine (mg)	53	62	50	0
Vitamins				
Vitamin A (IU)	8040	9720	5520	780
Vitamin D (IU)	2211	2675	1220	260
Vitamin E (IU)	31	36	32	3.4
Vitamin C (mg)	234	276	300	24
Thiamine (mg)	1.68	2	2	.187
Riboflavin (mg)	2.3	2.8	5.0	.25
Niacin (mg)	27	32	41	3.1
Vitamin B_6 (mg)	1.7	2.0	2	.19
Folacin (mcg)	234	276	300	23
Vitamin B_{12} (mcg)	2	2.4	4.5	.21
Vitamin K (mcg)	87	103	97	9.1
Pantothenic Acid (mg)	8.0	9.5	15	.8
Biotin (mcg)	13.4	15.8	300	.81
Osmolality mOsm/kg water	244	300	300	65
Renal Solute Load mOsm/liter	121	220	149	54

APPENDIX G (Continued)
NUTRIENT COMPOSITION OF COMMERCIAL INFANT FORMULAS

Infant Formulas: Full Term, Milk Based

Nutrient/liter	Full Term Human Milk	Enfamil 20	Similac 20	Similac 24	SMA 20	Similac PM 60/40
kcal/mL	0.68	0.67	0.67	0.8	0.67	0.67
Protein (g) (% total calories)	11 (6)	15 (9)	15 (9)	22 (11)	15 (9)	16 (9)
Source	whey/casein 60:40	whey/casein 60:40	whey/casein 18:82	whey/casein 18:82	whey/casein 60:40	whey/casein 60:40
Fat (g) (% total calories)	39 (52)	38 (50)	36.3 (48)	43 (47)	36 (48)	37.6 (50)
Source	human	45% soy oil 55% coconut oil	60% soy oil 40% coconut oil	60% soy oil 40% coconut oil	coconut, safflower, soy oils, oleo	60% soy oil 40% coconut oil
Carbohydrate (g) (% total calories)	72 (42)	69 (41)	72.3 (43)	85 (42)	72 (43)	69 (41)
(Source)	lactose	lactose	lactose	lactose	lactose	lactose
Water (g)	880	897	900	885	904	910
Mineral						
Calcium (mg) (mEq)	280 (14)	460 (23.0)	510 (25.0)	730 (37)	420 (20.9)	380 (19)
Phosphorus (mg)	150	315	390	570	280	190
Sodium (mg) (mEq)	180 (8)	180 (7.9)	190 (8)	280 (12)	150 (6.4)	160 (7)
Potassium (mg) (mEq)	530 (14)	724 (18.6)	730 (19)	1100 (29)	560 (14.3)	580 (15)
Chloride (mg) (mEq)	385 (11)	415 (11.8)	450 (13)	660 (19)	375 (10.6)	400 (11)
Magnesium (mg) (mEq)	40 (3.3)	52 (4.3)	41 (3.4)	57 (4.7)	45 (3.6)	41 (3.4)
Iron (mg)	0.3	12.7	12	15	12	1.5
Zinc (mg)	1.5	5.2	5.1	6.1	5	5.1
Copper (mg)	0.24	0.63	0.61	0.73	0.47	0.61
Manganese (mg)	0.006	0.10	0.03	0.04	0.15	0.34
Iodine (mg)	0.11	68	100	120	60	40
Vitamins						
Vitamin A (IU)	2200	2080	2030	2440	2000	2030
Vitamin D (IU)	22	415	410	490	400	410
Vitamin E (IU)	1.8	21	20	24	9.5	20
Vitamin C (mg)	50	55	60	70	55	60
Thiamine (mg)	0.21	0.52	0.68	0.81	0.67	0.68
Riboflavin (mg)	0.36	1.05	1.01	1.22	1.00	1.01
Niacin (mg)	1.83	8.4	7.1	8.5	5.0	7.1
Vitamin B_6 (mg)	0.205	0.42	0.41	0.49	0.42	0.41
Folacin (mcg)	52	104.5	100	120	50	100
Vitamin B_{12} (mcg)	0.3	1.6	1.7	2.0	1.3	1.7
Vitamin K (mcg)	2.1	57.6	54	65	55	54
Pantothenic Acid (mg)	1.8	3.15	3.04	3.65	2.1	3.04
Biotin (mcg)	4	15.4	30	36	15	30
Osmolality mOsm/kg water	300	300	300	380	300	280
Renal Solute Load mOsm/liter	73	97	100	146	91	95

NUTRIENT COMPOSITION OF COMMERCIAL
PEDIATRIC AND INFANT FORMULAS

Nutrient/liter	Full Term, Soy Based			Hypoallergenic Protein Hydrolysate		Modified Fat Source	Pediatric
	Pro-Sobee	Isomil	Nursoy	Nutramigen	Pregestimil	Portagen	Pediasure
kcal/mL	0.67	0.67	0.67	0.67	0.67	0.67	1.0
Protein (g) (% total calories)	20 (12)	18 (11)	21 (12)	19 (11)	19 (11)	23 (13)	30 (12)
Source	soy protein isolate & L-methionine	soy protein isolate & L-methionine	soy protein isolate	casein hydrolysate & L-cystine, L-tyrosine, L-tryptophan	casein hydrolysate & L-cystine L-tyrosine, L-tryptophan	casein	whey/casein 18:82
Fat (g) (% total calories)	36 (48)	37 (49)	36 (47)	26 (35)	27 (36)	32 (42)	49.7 (44)
Source	coconut & corn oils lactose	40% coconut & 60% soy oils	oleo, coconut, safflower & soy bean oil	corn oil 85 (42)	40% MCT, 60% corn oil	83% MCT 12% corn oil, 3% lecithin	50% safflower oil, 30% soy oil, 20% MCT
Carbohydrate (g)	67 (40)	68 (40)	69 (41)	90 (54)	90 (54)	77 (45)	110 (44)
Source	corn syrup & solids	corn syrup sucrose & modified cornstarch	sucrose	corn syrup solids & modified starch	corn syrup solids & modified tapioca starch	corn syrup solids & sucrose	hydrolyzed cornstarch, sucrose
Water (g)	898	900	898	898	900	898	845
Mineral							
Calcium (mg) (mEq)	630 (31.5)	710 (35.5)	600 (29.9)	630 (31.5)	630 (31.5)	630 (31.5)	970 (48.4)
Phosphorus (mg)	496	507	420	415	415	470	800
Sodium (mg) (mEq)	241 (10.5)	318 (13.8)	200 (8.7)	315 (13.6)	315 (13.6)	368 (16)	380 (16.5)
Potassium (mg) (mEq)	819 (21)	730 (18.2)	700 (17.9)	730 (18.8)	730 (18.8	837 (21.5)	1305 (33.5)
Chloride (mg) (mEq)	556 (15.7)	439 (12.3)	375 (10.6)	576 (16)	576 (16)	576 (16)	1010 (28.6)
Magnesium (mg) (mEq)	73 (6.1)	50 (4.2)	67	74 (6.1)	74 (6.1)	134 (11.2)	200 (16.6)
Iron (mg)	12.6	12.2	11.5	12.7	12.7	12.7	14
Zinc (mg)	5.2	5.0	5.0	5.2	4.2	6.3	12
Copper (mg)	0.63	0.50	0.47	0.63	0.63	1.05	1.0
Manganese (mg)	0.17	0.20	0.20	0.21	0.21	0.85	2.5
Iodine (mcg)	68	100	60	48	47	47	95
Vitamins							
Vitamin A (IU)	2080	2010	2000	2080	2080	5230	2570
Vitamin D (IU)	415	402	400	415	415	525	505
Vitamin E (IU)	21	20	9.5	16	16	21	21
Vitamin C (mg)	54.3	60.3	55	54.3	54.3	54.3	100
Thiamine (mg)	0.52	0.40	0.67	0.52	.52	1.0	2.7
Riboflavin (mg)	0.63	0.60	100	0.63	0.63	1.26	2.1
Niacin (mg)	8.4	9.0	5.0	8.4	8.4	14.1	16.5
Vitamin B_6 (mg)	0.42	0.40	0.42	0.42	0.42	1.4	2.6
Folacin (mcg)	105	101	50	105	105	105	370
Vitamin B_{12} (mcg)	2.1	3.0	2.0	2.1	2.1	4.2	6
Vitamin K (mcg)	105	101	100	105	105	105	34
Pantothenic Acid (mg)	3.1	5.0	3.0	3.1	3.1	7.0	10
Biotin (mcg)	52.3	30.2	35	52.5	52.3	52.3	320
Osmolality mOsm/kg water	200	240	296	320	350	220	325
Renal Solute Load mOsm/liter	130	116	122	126	125	147	200

TUBE FEEDING SUPPLEMENTS AVAILABLE AT UNIVERSITY OF MICHIGAN HOSPITALS

A. Electrolytes

1. Calcium: Titralac® 1000 mg/5 mL provides 400 mg elemental calcium (20 mEq) as carbonate salt
2. Magnesium*: 400 mg tablet provides 240 mg elemental magnesium (10 mEq) as oxide salt
3. Phosphate: Neutra-phos capsule provides 250 mg elemental phosphorus (8mM) as sodium, potassium salt

B. Minerals

1. Zinc*: 220 mg tablet provides 50 mg elemental zinc as sulfate salt

C. Vitamin Preparations

Name Dosage	Vit A (IU)	D (IU)	E (IU)	B_1 (mg)	B_2 (mg)	Niacin (mg)	PA+ (mg)	B_6 (mg)	B_{12} (mcg)	C (mg)	Biotin (mcg)	FA** (mcg)	Fe (mg)	Flouride (mg)
Poly-Vi-Sol® 1 mL dose***	1500	400	5	0.5	0.6	8	—	0.4	2	35	—	—	—	—
Bugs Bunny Flinstone® Chewable Tablets*	2500	400	15	1.05	1.2	13.5	—	1.05	4.5	60	—	300	—	—
Tri-Vi-Flor® 1 mL dose***	1500	400	—	—	—	—	—	—	—	35	—	—	—	0.25

D. Carbohydrate, Fat and Protein Modular Component

Polycose®	2.0 kcal/mL	500 g CHO/liter
Microlipid®	4.5 kcal/mL	500 g fat/liter
MCT oil®	7.7 kcal/mL	933 g fat/liter
Propac®	4.0 kcal/g	15 g pro/19.5 g
Duocal®	4.7 kcal/g	22 g fat, 73 g CHO/100 g

*Crushable   +Pantothenic Acid   **Folic Acid   ***Pediatric dose: 1 mL / Adult dose: 2 mL

APPENDIX I

NUTRIENT COMPOSITION OF ORAL FORMULAS PREPARED BY THE DEPARTMENT OF DIETETICS AT THE UNIVERSITY OF MICHIGAN HOSPITALS

Name	Caloric Density (kcal/mL)	Composition (Source) Carbohydrate (g/L)	Protein (g/L)	Fat (g/L)	Ingredients	Electrolytes (mEq/100 mL) Na	K	Characteristics and Usage
Whole milk	.653	47 mg/L (29% of kcal)	33 g/L (20% of kcal)	37 g/L (51% of kcal)		2.2	3.9	*Contains lactose
Milkshake	1.3	142 g/L (44% of kcal)	37.5 g/L (12% of kcal)	62.5 g/L (44% of kcal)	Ice cream, whole milk, skim milk powder, flavoring	3.1	4.8	*Contains lactose; chocolate, strawberry, vanilla flavors
Creamy milkshakes (Average)	2.6	104 g/L (16% of kcal)	62 g/L (9% of kcal)	217 g/L (75% of kcal)	Whipping cream, ice cream, egg white powder, sugar	4.4	3.7	*Contains lactose; high calorie; chocolate, strawberry, vanilla
Peanut butter drink	3.3	183 g/L (22% of kcal)	58 g/L (7% of kcal)	262 g/L (71% of kcal)	Heavy whipping cream, smooth peanut butter, ice cream, chocolate syrup	5.9	5.0	*Contains lactose;
Hawaiian punch citrotein	.9	196 g/L (87% of kcal)	29 g/L (13% of kcal)	0	Hawaiian punch, citrotein	3.1	2.0	Clear liquid, lowfat protein source
Lemonade citrotein	.7	142 g/L (83% of kcal)	29 g/L (17% of kcal)	0	Lemonade, citrotein	2.3	1.5	Clear liquid, lowfat protein source
Meritene (Average)	.9	108 g/L (44% of kcal)	62 g/L (25% of kcal)	33 g/L (31% of kcal)	Meritene, whole milk	4.3	6.9	*Contains lactose; chocolate, vanilla
Swiss Miss Drink	1.8	246 g/L (55% of kcal)	50 g/L (11% of kcal)	67 g/L (34% of kcal)	Milk, ice cream, chocolate mix, egg nog base	4.9	4.9	*Contains lactose chocolate flavored

APPENDIX J
RECOMMENDED DIETARY ALLOWANCES

	Age (years)	Weight (kg)	Weight (lbs)	Height (cm)	Height (in)	Protein (g)	Vitamin A (mcg RE)[3]	Vitamin D (mcg)[4]	Vitamin E (mg or TE)[5]	Vitamin K (mcg)	Vitamin C (mg)	Thiamine (mg)
Infants	0.0-0.5	6	13	60	24	13	375	7.5	3	5	30	0.3
	0.5-1.0	9	20	71	28	14	375	10	4	10	35	0.4
Children	1-3	13	29	90	35	16	400	10	6	15	40	0.7
	4-6	20	44	112	44	24	500	10	7	20	45	0.9
	7-10	28	62	132	52	28	700	10	7	30	45	1.0
Males	11-14	45	99	157	62	45	1000	10	10	45	50	1.3
	15-18	66	145	176	69	59	1000	10	10	65	60	1.5
	19-24	72	160	177	70	58	1000	10	10	70	60	1.5
	25-50	79	174	176	70	63	1000	10	10	80	60	1.5
	51+	77	170	173	68	63	1000	5	10	80	60	1.2
Females	11-14	46	101	157	62	46	800	10	8	45	50	1.1
	15-18	55	120	163	64	44	800	10	8	55	60	1.1
	19-24	58	128	164	65	46	800	10	8	60	60	1.1
	25-50	63	138	163	64	50	800	5	8	65	60	1.1
	51+	65	143	160	63	50	800	5	8	65	60	1.0
Pregnant						60	800	10	10	65	70	1.5
Lactating	1st 6 mo.					65	1300	10	12	65	95	1.6
	2nd 6 mo.					62	1200	10	11	65	90	1.6

Fat-Soluble Vitamins: Vitamin A, Vitamin D, Vitamin E, Vitamin K. Water-Soluble Vitamins: Vitamin C, Thiamine.

APPENDIX J (Continued)
RECOMMENDED DIETARY ALLOWANCES

	Age Years	Riboflavin (mg)	Niacin (mg NE)[6]	Vitamin B$_6$ (mg)	Folacin[2] (mcg)	Vitamin B$_{12}$ (mcg)	Calcium (mg)	Phosphorus (mg)	Magnesium (mg)	Iron (mg)	Zinc (mg)	Iodine (mcg)	Selenium (mcg)
Infants	0.0-0.5	0.4	5	0.3	25	0.3[a]	400	300	40	6	5	40	10
	0.5-1.0	0.5	6	0.6	35	0.5	600	500	60	10	5	50	15
Children	1-3	0.8	9	1.0	50	0.7	800	800	80	10	10	70	20
	4-6	1.1	12	1.1	75	1.0	800	800	120	10	10	90	20
	7-10	1.2	13	1.4	100	1.4	800	800	170	10	10	120	30
Males	11-14	1.5	17	1.7	150	2.0	1200	1200	270	12	15	150	40
	15-18	1.8	20	2.0	200	2.0	1200	1200	400	12	15	150	50
	19-24	1.7	19	2.0	200	2.0	1200	1200	350	10	15	150	70
	25-50	1.7	19	2.0	200	2.0	800	800	350	10	15	150	70
	51+	1.4	15	2.0	200	2.0	800	800	350	10	15	150	70
Females	11-14	1.3	15	1.4	150	2.0	1200	1200	280	15	12	150	45
	15-18	1.3	15	1.5	180	2.0	1200	1200	300	15	12	150	50
	19-24	1.3	15	1.6	180	2.0	1200	1200	280	15	12	150	55
	25-50	1.3	15	1.6	180	2.0	800	800	280	15	12	150	55
	51+	1.2	13	1.6	180	2.0	800	800	280	10	12	150	55
Pregnant		1.6	17	2.2	400	2.2	1200	1200	320	30	15	175	65
Lactating	1st 6 mo.	1.8	20	2.1	280	2.6	1200	1200	355	15	19	200	75
	2nd 6 mo.	1.7	20	2.1	260	2.6	1200	1200	340	15	16	200	75

Food and Nutrition Board, National Academy of Sciences—National Research Council Recommended Dietary Allowances, Revised 1989.

1. The allowances are intended to provide for individual variations among most normal persons as they live in the United States under usual environmental stresses. Diets should be based on a variety of common foods to provide other nutrients for which human requirements have been less well defined.

2. The folacin allowances refer to dietary sources as determined by Lactobacillus casei assay after treatment with enzymes ("conjugates") to make polyglutamyl forms of the vitamin available to the test organism.

3. Retinol equivalents. 1 Retinol equivalent = 1 mcg retinol or 6 mcg carotene.

4. As cholecalciferol 10 mcg cholecalciferol = 400 IU vitamin D.

5. or tocopherol equivalents. 1 mcg d-or-tocopherol = 1 or T.E.

6. 1 N E (niacin equivalent) is equal to mg of niacin or 60 mcg of dietary tryptophan.

a The RDA for vitamin B$_{12}$ in infants is based on average concentration of the vitamin in human milk. The allowances after weaning are based on energy intake (as recommended by the American Academy of Pediatrics) and consideration of other factors such as intestinal absorption.

APPENDIX K

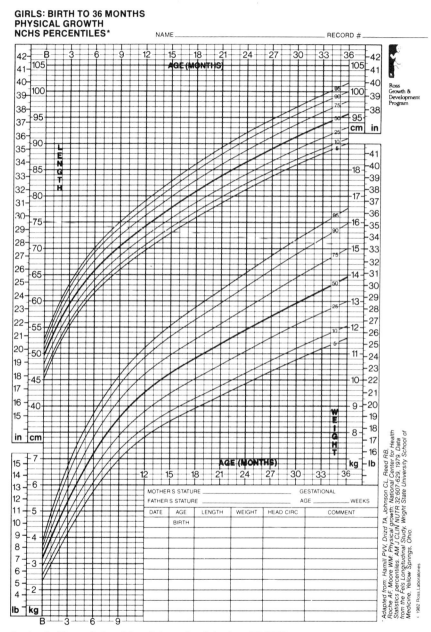

GIRLS: BIRTH TO 36 MONTHS
PHYSICAL GROWTH
NCHS PERCENTILES*

NAME _____ RECORD # _____

Ross
Growth &
Development
Program

MOTHER'S STATURE _____ GESTATIONAL

FATHER'S STATURE _____ AGE _____ WEEKS

DATE	AGE	LENGTH	WEIGHT	HEAD CIRC	COMMENT
	BIRTH				

*Adapted from: Hamill PVV, Drizd TA, Johnson CL, Reed RB, Roche AF, Moore WM. Physical growth: National Center for Health Statistics percentiles. AM J CLIN NUTR 32:607-629, 1979. Data from the Fels Longitudinal Study, Wright State University School of Medicine, Yellow Springs, Ohio.

© 1982 Ross Laboratories

Reprinted with permission of Ross Laboratories, Columbus, OH 43216

APPENDIX K (Continued)

**GIRLS: BIRTH TO 36 MONTHS
PHYSICAL GROWTH
NCHS PERCENTILES***

NAME_____ RECORD # _____

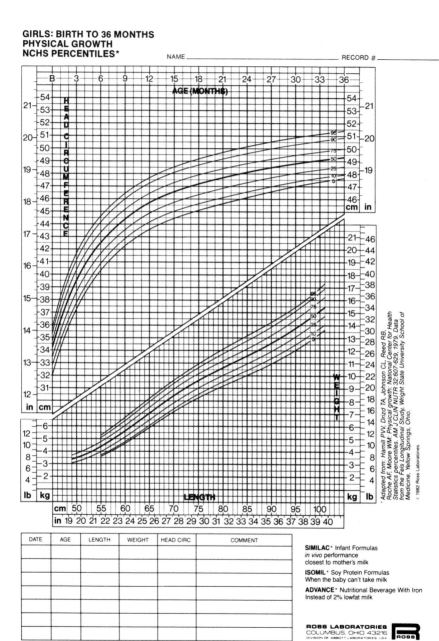

DATE	AGE	LENGTH	WEIGHT	HEAD CIRC	COMMENT

SIMILAC* Infant Formulas
in vivo performance
closest to mother's milk

ISOMIL* Soy Protein Formulas
When the baby can't take milk

ADVANCE* Nutritional Beverage With Iron
Instead of 2% lowfat milk

ROSS LABORATORIES
COLUMBUS, OHIO 43216
DIVISION OF ABBOTT LABORATORIES USA

G106(0 05) JANUARY 1986   LITHO IN USA

Reprinted with permission of Ross Laboratories, Columbus, OH 43216

* Adapted from: Hamill PVV, Drizd TA, Johnson CL, Reed RB, Roche AF, Moore WM: Physical growth: National Center for Health Statistics percentiles. AM J CLIN NUTR 32:607-629, 1979. Data from the Fels Longitudinal Study, Wright State University School of Medicine, Yellow Springs, Ohio.

© 1982 Ross Laboratories

APPENDIX K (Continued)

BOYS: BIRTH TO 36 MONTHS
PHYSICAL GROWTH
NCHS PERCENTILES*

NAME _____ RECORD # _____

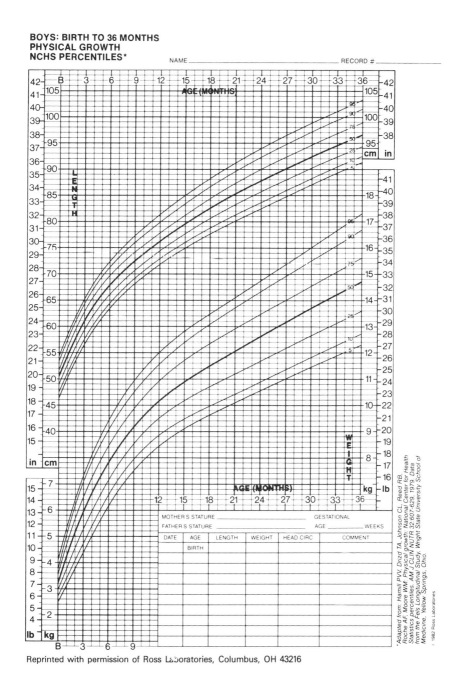

Reprinted with permission of Ross Laboratories, Columbus, OH 43216

*Adapted from Hamill PVV, Drizd TA, Johnson CL, Reed RB, Roche AF, Moore WM. Physical growth: National Center for Health Statistics percentiles. AM J CLIN NUTR 32:607-629, 1979. Data from the Fels Longitudinal Study, Wright State University School of Medicine, Yellow Springs, Ohio.

© 1982 Ross Laboratories

APPENDIX K (Continued)

BOYS: BIRTH TO 36 MONTHS
PHYSICAL GROWTH
NCHS PERCENTILES*

NAME _____ RECORD # _____

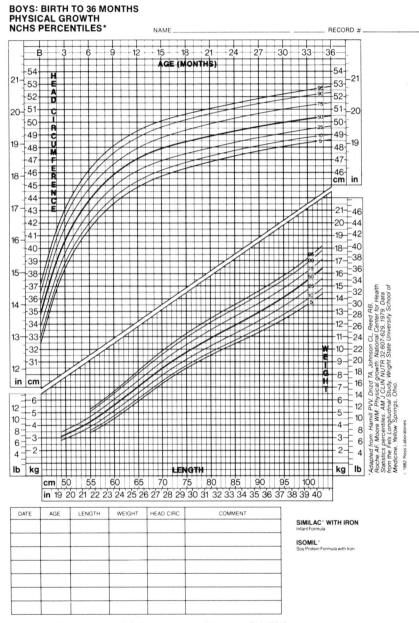

DATE	AGE	LENGTH	WEIGHT	HEAD CIRC	COMMENT

SIMILAC® WITH IRON
Infant Formula

ISOMIL®
Soy Protein Formula with Iron

Reprinted with permission of Ross Laboratories, Columbus, OH 43216

104

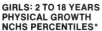

GIRLS: 2 TO 18 YEARS
PHYSICAL GROWTH
NCHS PERCENTILES*

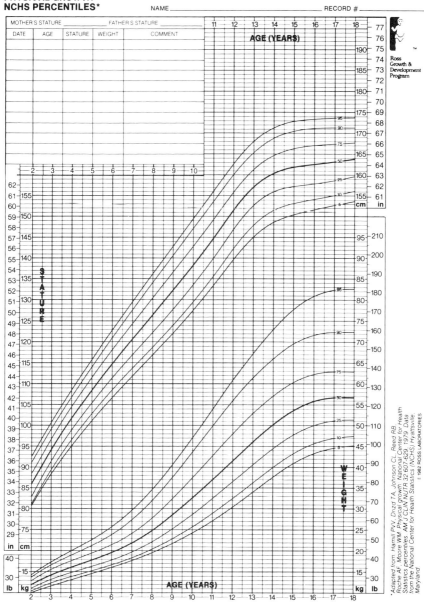

Reprinted with permission of Ross Laboratories, Columbus, OH 43216

APPENDIX K (Continued)

GIRLS: PREPUBESCENT
PHYSICAL GROWTH
NCHS PERCENTILES*

NAME _____ RECORD # _____

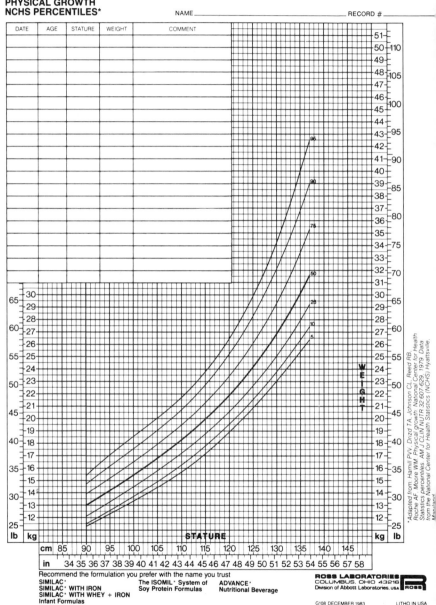

Reprinted with permission of Ross Laboratories, Columbus, OH 43216

APPENDIX K (Continued)

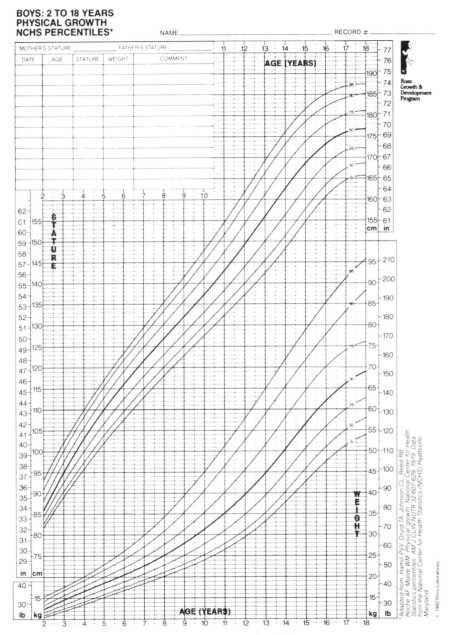

BOYS: 2 TO 18 YEARS
PHYSICAL GROWTH
NCHS PERCENTILES*

NAME _____ RECORD # _____

Ross
Growth &
Development
Program

AGE (YEARS)

STATURE

WEIGHT

*Adapted from Hamill PVV, Drizd TA, Johnson CL, Reed RB Roche AF, Moore WM. Physical growth: National Center for Health Statistics percentiles. AM J CLIN NUTR 32:607-629, 1979. Data from the National Center for Health Statistics (NCHS) Hyattsville, Maryland

Reprinted with permission of Ross Laboratories, Columbus, OH 43216

APPENDIX K (Continued)

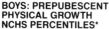

BOYS: PREPUBESCENT PHYSICAL GROWTH NCHS PERCENTILES*

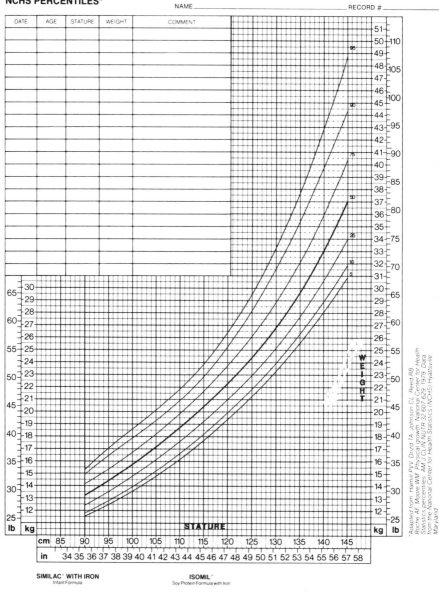

BIBLIOGRAPHY AND SELECTED READINGS GENERAL REVIEW

GENERAL

A.S.P.E.N. Board of Directors Guidelines for Use of Total Parenteral Nutrition in the Hospitalized Adult Patient. JPEN 10:441, 1986.

Deitel, Mervyn (ed): Nutrition in Clinical Surgery (second edition), Williams & Wilkins, Baltimore, 1985.

Fischer JE (ed): Surgical Nutrition, Little, Brown & Co. Boston, 1983.

Goodhart RS and Shils ME (eds): Modern nutrition in health and disease, Lea and Febiger, Philadelphia, 1980.

Jeejeebhoy KN (ed): Total Parenteral Nutrition in the Hospital and Home, CRC Press, Boca Raton, 1983.

Johnston IDA (ed): Advances in Clinical Nutrition, MTP Press, Boston 1983.

Kirkpatrick JR (ed): Nutrition and Metabolism in the Surgical Patient, Futura Publishing Co, Mount Kisco, 1983.

Linder MC (ed): Nutritional Biochemistry and Metabolism, Elsevier, N.Y., 1985.

Nehme AE: Nutritional support of the hospitalized patient. The Team Concept, JAMA 243:1906, 1980.

Pike RL and Brown mL (eds): Nutrition, An Integrated Approach (third ed), J. Wiley and Sons, N.Y., 1984.

Rombeau JL and Caldwell MD (eds): Parenteral Nutrition, W.B. Saunders, Philadelphia, 1986.

Suskind RM (ed): Textbook of Pediatric Nutrition, Raven Press, New York, 1981.

ADDITIVES

American Medical Association: AMA guidelines for essential trace element preparations for parenteral use, JPEN 3:263, 1979.

American Medical Association Department of Foods and Nutrition, 1975: AMA guidelines for multivitamin preparations, JPEN 3:258, 1979.

Allison R: Plasma trace elements during total parenteral nutrition, JPEN 2:35, 1978.

Bailey MJ: Reduction of catheter-associated sepsis in parenteral nutrition using low-dose intravenous heparin, Br Med J 1:1671, 1979.

Crasad AS (ed): Clinical Biochemical, and Nutritional Aspects of Trace Elements, Alan R. Liss, Inc, New York, 1982.

Eggert LD, Rusho WJ, MacKay et al: Calcium and phosphorus compatibility in parenteral nutrition solutions for neonates, Am J Hosp Pharm 39:49, 1982.

Mirtallo JM, Rogers KR, Johnson JA et al: Stability of amino acids and the availability of acid in total parenteral nutrition solutions containing hydrochloric.

O'Dwyer ST, Smith RT, H Wang TL, Willmore DW: Maintenance of small bowel mucosa with glutamine enriched parenteral nutrition, JPEN 13:599, 1989.

Rennert OM and Chan WY: Metabolism of trace elements in man, CRC Press, Boca Raton, 1984.

Shaw JC: Trace elements in the fetus and young infant I. Zinc, Am J Dis Child 133:1260, 1979.

Shaw JC: Trace elements in the fetus and young infant II. Copper, manganese, selenium, and chromium, Am J Dis Child 134:74, 1980.

Wan KK and Tsallas G: Dilute iron dextran formulation for addition to parenteral nutrient solutions, Am J Hosp Pharm 37:206, 1980.

Weber SS, Wood WA, Jackson EA: Availability of insulin from parenteral nutrient solutions, Am J Hosp Pharm 34:353, 1977.

COMPLICATIONS

Askanazi J, Rosenbaum SH, Hyman AI et al: Respiratory changes induced by the large glucose loads of total parenteral nutrition, JAMA 243:1444, 1980.

Askanazi J, Elwyn DH, Silverberg PA et al: Respiratory distress secondary to a high carbohydrate load: a case report, Surgery 87:596, 1980.

Benjamin DR: Hepatobiliary dysfunction in infants and children associated with long term total parenteral nutrition. A clinicopathologic study, Am J Clin Pathol 76:276, 1981.

Cerra F: Hypermetabolism, organ failure and metabolic support. Surgery 101:1-14, 1987.

Faubion WC, Bollish SJ, Wesley JR: Central venous catheter occlusion treated by thrombolytic agents, NSS 3:2, 1983.

Faubion WC, Wesley, JR, Khalidi N, Silva J: TPN catheter sepsis: impact of the team approach, JPEN 10:642, 1986.

Knapke CM, Owens JP, Mirtallo JM: Management of glucose abnormalities in patients receiving total parenteral nutrition, Clin Pharm 8:136, 1989.

Grant JP: Subclavian catheter insertion and complications, Handbook of parenteral nutrition, WB Saunders and Co, Philadelphia, p. 47, 1980.

Khalidi N, Wesley JR, Thoene JG et al: Biotin deficiency in a patient with short bowel syndrome during home parenteral nutrition, JPEN 8:311-114, 1984.

Kovacevich D, Faubion WC, Bender J et al: Association of PN catheter sepsis with urinary tract infections, JPEN 10:639-41, 1986.

Mack DM, de Lorimer AA, Liebman WM et al: Biotin deficiency: an unusual complication of parenteral alimentation, N Engl J Med 304:820, 1981.

Maki DG, Weise CE, Sarafin HW: A semiquantitative culture method for identifying intravenous-catheter-related infection, N Engl J Med 296:1305, 1977.

Sheldon GF and Baker C: Complications of nutritional support, Crit Care Med 8:35, 1980.

Shike M, Sturtridge WC, Tam CS et al: A possible role of vitamin D in the genesis of parenteral nutrition induced metabolic bone disease, Ann Intern Med 95:560, 1981.

Solomon SM, Kirby DF: The refeeding syndrome: a review, JPEN 14:90, 1990.

Wakefield A, Cohen Z, Craig M et al: Thrombogenicity of total parenteral nutritional solutions: I. effect on induction of monocyte/macrophage procoagulant activity, Gastroenterology 97:1210, 1989.

Weisner RL and Krumdieck CL: Death resulting from overzealous total parenteral nutrition: the refeeding syndrome revisited, Am J Clin Nutr 34:393, 1980.

ENTERAL — Adult and Pediatric

Anderson SA, Chin HI, Fisher KD: History and current status of infant formulas, AJCN 25:381-397, 1982.

Andrassy RJ, Page CP et al: Continual catheter administration of an elemental diet in infants and children, Surg Nutr 82;205-210, 1977.

Brady MS, Rickard KA et al: Formulas and human milk for premature infants; A review and update, JADA 81:547-555, 1982.

Cataidi-Betcher EM et al: Complications occurring during enteral nutrition support: A prospective study, JPEN 7(6):546-552, 1983.

Ford E, Jennings L, Andrassy R, Serum albumin (oncotic pressure) correlates with enteral feeding tolerance in the pediatric surgical patient. J Ped Surg 22:597-9, 1987.

Heimburger DC and Weinsier RL: Guidelines for evaluating and categorizing enteral feeding formulas according to therapeutic equivalence, JPEN 9:61, 1985.

LeLeiko NS, Murray C, Munro HN: Enteral Support of the hospitalized child. In Suskind R (ed): Textbook of Pediatric Nutrition, New York, Raven Press, p. 357, 1981.

Randali HT: Enteral Nutrition: Tube feeding in acute and chronic illness, JPEN 8:113-136, 1984.

Rombeau JL and Caldwell MD (eds): Enteral and Tube Feeding, Clinical Nutrition, WB Saunders, Philadelphia, 1984.

Ryan SA and Page CB: Intrajejunal feeding: Development and current status, JPEN 8:187, 1984.

FAT EMULSION AND ESSENTIAL FATT ACID DEFICIENCY

Adamkin DH, Gelke KN, Andrews BF, Fat emulsion and hypertriglyceridemia, JPEN 8:563-567, 1984.

American Academy of Pediatrics Committee on Nutrition, Use of intravenous fat emulsions in pediatric patients, Pediatrics 618:738, 1981.

Andrew G, Chan G, Schiff D: Lipid metabolism in the neonate I. The effects of Intralipid® infusion on plasma triglyceride and free fatty acid concentrations in the neonate, J Pediatr 88:273, 1976.

Andrew G, Chan G, Schiff D: Lipid metabolism in the neonate II. The effect of Intralipid® infusion in the neonate, J Pediatr 92:995, 1978.

Bark S, Holm I, Hakansson I: Nitrogen sparing effect of fat emulsion compared with glucose in the postoperative period, Acta Chir Scand 142:423, 1976.

Friedman Z: Essential fatty acids revisited, Am J Dis Child, 134:397, 1980.

Plim A, Carnielli V, Tiller RM, Smith J, Heim T: Metabolism of intravenous fat emulsion in the surgical newborn, J Ped Surg 24:95, 1989.

Shennan AT, Bryan MH, Angel A: The effect of gestational age on Intralipid® tolerance in newborn infants, J Pediatr 91:134, 1977.

HOME PN

Bender JM, Faubion WC: Parenteral nutrition for the pediatric patient, Home Health Care Nurse 3:6,32, 1985.

Dudrick SJ, Englert DM, Van Buren CT et al: New concepts of ambulatory home hyperalimentation JPEN 3:72, 1979.

Jeejeebhoy KN, Langer B, Tsallas G et al: Total parenteral nutrition at home: studies in patients surviving 4 months to 5 years, Gastroenterology 71:943, 1976.

Lees CD, Steiger E, Hooley RA et al: Home parenteral nutrition, Surg Clin North Am 61:621, 1981.

Pollak PF, Kadden M, Byrne WJ et al: 100 patient years' experience with the Broviac silastic catheter for central venous nutrition, JPEN 5, 32-36, 1981.

Wesley JR, Home parenteral nutrition: indications, principles, and cost-effectiveness, Comprehensive Therapy 9:29-36, 1983.

Wesley JR, Khalidi N, Faubion WC et al: Home parenteral nutrition: A hospital based program with commercial logistic support, JPEN 8:585, 1984.

LIVER DYSFUNCTION AND BRANCHED CHAIN AMINO ACID THERAPY

Blackburn GL, Moldawer LL, Sadahito U et al: Branched chain amino acid administration and metabolism during starvation, injury and infection, Surgery 86:307, 1979.

Bower RH and Fischer JE: Nutritional management of hepatic encephalopathy, Adv Nutr Res 5:1, 1983.

Fischer JE and Baldessarini RJ: False neurotransmitters and hepatic failure, Lancet 2:75, 1971.

Fischer JE, Rosen HM, Ebeird AM et al: The effect of normalization of plasma amino acids in hepatic encephalopathy in man, Surgery 80:70, 1976.

Freund HR, Yoshimura N, Fischer JE: Chronic hepatic encephalopathy, long-term therapy with a branched chain amino-acid-enriched elemental diet, JAMA 242:347, 1979.

James JH, Jeppson B, Ziparo V et al. Hyperammonemia, plasma amino acid imbalance, and blood-brain amino acid transport: A unified theory of portal-systemic encephalopathy, Lancet 2:772, 1979.

Lindor KD, Fleming CR, Abrams A: Liver function values in adults receiving total parenteral nutrition, JAMA 241:2398, 1979.

Rosen HM, Yoshimura N, Hodgman JM et al: Plasma amino acid patterns in hepatic encephalopathy of differing etiology, Gastroenterology 72:483, 1977.

Sheldon GF, Peterson SR, Sanders R: Hepatic dysfunction during hyperalimentation, Arch Surg 113:504, 1978.

Striebel JP, Holm E, Lutz HE et al: Parenteral nutrition and coma therapy with amino acids in hepatic failure, JPEN 3:240, 1979.

MALIGNANT DISEASE

Bozzette, Federico: Effects of Artificial Nutrition on the Nutrition Staus of Cancer Patients. JPEN 13:406, 1989.

Brennan MF: Total parenteral nutrition in the cancer patient, N Engl J Med 305:375, 1981.

Burt ME, Stein TP, Schwade JG, Brennan MF: Effects of total parenteral nutrition on protein metabolism in man, AJCN 34:628, 1981.

Daly JM, Dudrick SJ, Copeland EM III, Effect on delayed cutaneous hypersensitivity in cancer patients, Ann Surg 192:587, 1980.

Mullin TJ and Kirkpatrick JR: The effect of nutritional support on immune competency in patients suffering from trauma, sepsis, or malignant disease, Surgery 90:610, 1981.

Ota DM, Copeland EM III, Corriere JN Jr, Dudrick SJ: The effects of nutrition and treatment of cancer on host immunocompetence, Surg Gyncol Obstet 148:104, 1979.

Steffee WP and Krey SH: Enteral hyperalimentation of the cancer patient, Newell GR and Ellison NM (eds): Nutrition and cancer: Etiology and treatment, Ravin Press, New York, 1981.

NUTRITIONAL ASSESSMENT

Detsky A, Baker J, Mendelson R, et al, Evaluating the accuracy of nutritional assessment techniques applied to hospitalized patients: methodology and comparisons. JPEN 8:153, 1984.

Kaminiski M and Jeejeebhoy K: Nutritional assessment-diagnosis of malnutrition and selection of therapy, J Surg Prac 8:45, 1979.

McLaren DA and Mequed MM: Nutritional assessment at the crossroads, JPEN 7(6):575, 1983.

Miller SF: Nutritional assessment and support: Scientific inquiry, Journal of Trauma 23:68, 1983.

Solomons NW and Allen LH: The functional assessment of nutritional status: Principles, practice and potential, Nutr Rev 41:33, 1983.

Starker PM, Gump FE et al: Serum albumin levels as an index of nutritional support, Surgery 9:194, 1982.

Steffee WP: Malnutrition in hospitalized patients, JAMA 244:26, 1980.

Stromberg BV, Davis RJ, Danzeger LH: Relationship of serum transferrin to total iron binding capacity for nutritional assessment, JPEN 6:392-394, 1982.

Wilmore DW: The metabolic management of the critically ill, Plenum Medical Book, New York, 1977.

PEDIATRICS

Andrassy RJ and Wolley MM: Progress in the use of elemental diets in infants and children, Surg Gynecol Obstet 147:701, 1978.

Benner JW, Coran AG, Weintraub WH, Wesley JR: The importance of different calorie sources in the intravenous nutrition of infants and children, Surgery 86:429, 1979.

Brans WY: Parenteral nutrition of the very low birth weight neonate: A critical view, Clin Perinatol 4:367, 1977.

Braunschweig CL, Wesley JR, Clark SF, Mercer NM: Rationale and guidelines for transitional feeding in the 3-30 kg child, JADA, (In Press).

Coran AG, Wesley JR: The pediatric patient, in Kirkpatrick JR (ed) Nutrition and metabolism in the surgical patient, Futura Publishing Co, Mount Kisco, 1983 pp. 445-482.

Dechert R, Wesley JR, Schafer L et al: Comparison of oxygen consumptions, carbon dioxide production, and resting energy expenditure in premature and full term infants, J Ped Surg 20:792, 1985.

Jacobs WC, Lazzara A, Martin DJ: Parenteral nutrition in the neonate, Abbott Laboratories, North Chicago, 1980.

Kerner JA, Manual of pediatric parenteral nutrition, John Wiley & Sons, New York, 1983.

LaMond S, Wesley JR, Dechert R et al, Correlation of cumulative calorie balance to weight gain in sick infants., JPEN 9:120, 1985.

Walker AW, Hendricks KM: Manual of pediatric nutrition, W.B. Saunders Co, Philadelphia, 1985.

PERIPHERAL NUTRITION

Bell EF, Walrburton D, Stonestreet BS: Effect of fluid administration on the development of symptomatic patient ductus arteriosus and congestive heart failure in premature infants, N Engl J Med 303:598, 1980.

Coran AG: Total intravenous feeding of infants and children without the use of a central venous catheter, Ann Surg 179:445, 1974.

Coran AG and Weintraub WH: Peripheral intravenous nutrition without fat in neonatal surgery, J Pediatr Surg 12:195, 1977.

Deitel M and Kaminsky V: Total nutrition by peripheral vein—the lipid system, Can Med Assoc J 11:154, 1974.

Jeejeebhoy KN, Anderson GH, Nakhooda AF et al: Metabolic studies in total parenteral nutrition with lipid in man-comparison with glucose, J Clin Invest 57:125, 1976.

Olson GB, Teasley KM, Cerra FB: Peripheral parenteral nutrition, Nutr Supp Serv 3:51, 1983.

Silberman H, Freehauf M, Fong G et al: Parenteral nutrition with lipids, JAMA 238:1380, 1977.

RENAL FAILURE AND ESSENTIAL AMINO ACID THERAPY

Abel RM: Nutritional support in the patient with acute renal failure, Journal of the American College of Nutrition 2:33, 1983.

Abel RM, Beck VE, Abbott WM et al: Improved survival from acute renal failure after treatment with intravenous essential amino acids and glucose, N Engl J Med 288:695, 1973.

Attman PO, Bucht H, Isaksson B, Uddenbom G: Nitrogen balance studies with amino acid supplemented low protein diet in uremia, Am J Clin Nutr 32:2033 1979.

Blackburn G, Etter G, MacKenzie T: Criteria for choosing amino acid therapy in acute renal failure, Am J Clin Nutr 31:1841, 1978.

Feinstein E, Blumenkrantz M, Heally M, Koffler A et al: Clinical and metabolic responses to parenteral nutrition in acute renal failure, Medicine 60:124, 1981.

First P and Ahlberg M: Principles of essential amino acid therapy in uremia, Am J Clin Nutr 31:1744, 1978.

Freund H, Atamian S, Fischer JE: Comparative study of parenteral nutrition in renal failure using essential and nonessential amino acid containing solutions, Surg Gynecol Obstet 151:652, 1980.

Leonard C, Luke R, Siegal R: Parenteral essential amino acids in acute renal failure, Urology, 6:154, 1975.

Steffee W: Nutritional support in renal failure, Surg Clin North Am 61:661, 1983.

Thurau K: Pathophysiology of the acutely failing kidney, Clinical Experimental Dialysis and Apheresis 7:9, 1983.

Wassner SJ, Sanders R, Orloff S et al: A comparison of essential and general amino acid infusions in protein depleted patients, Am J Clin Nutr 32:1497, 1979.

Wolk RA and Swartz RD: Nutritional support of patients with acute renal failure, Nutrition Support Services 6:38, 1986.